Be Your Own Beautician

Learn-it-Yourself Books are specially designed to enable the readers to learn useful skills and techniques, and obtain sound, authoritative information of value in their professional, family and personal lives.

The subjects of these books have been selected on the criterion of their utility for a large number of readers. The books are comprehensive and in some cases, are designed as work-books to serve the readers as self-learning guides.

Aroona Reejhsinghani, is perhaps the most prolific of Indian writers writing in English on subjects of interest to women readers. A dozen of her books have already been published and her numerous articles appear regulaıly in various magazines.

"...will be welcomed by the aware woman who is on the hunt for a simple but comprehensive guide." Femina

"...illustrates how our grandmothers' home made beauty-aids do not only vie with modern cosmetics but are pure and harmless - and also cheaper." Hindustan Times

Be your own beautician

Aroona Reejhsinghani

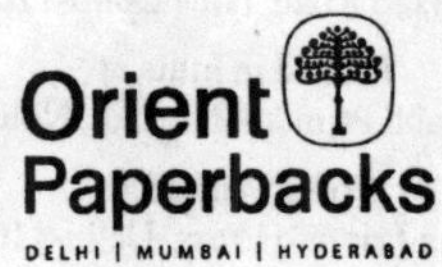

www.orientpaperbacks.com

ISBN 13: 978-81-222-0032-4
ISBN 10: 81-222-0032-X

1st Published 1976
14th Printing 2007

Be Your Own Beautician

Published by
Orient Paperbacks
(A division of Vision Books Pvt. Ltd.)
5A/8 Ansari Road, New Delhi-110 002

Printed in India at
Saurabh Printers Pvt. Ltd., Noida

Cover Printed at
Ravindra Printing Press, Delhi-110 006

Contents

Preface

SINCE TIMES immemorial, women have tried to improve upon nature by devising various ways and means to make themselves look more attractive. Our grandmothers did not have any beauty saloons where they could go for beauty treatment. They had to 'make do' with home-made remedies. These beauty aids, which have been handed down to us, are time-tested recipes, pure and harmless. Therefore, instead of wasting your time and money on expensive beauty saloons, try these home-brewed beauty aids and you will be surprised with the results.

It took me two years to complete this unique book, in the course of which I met a number of women who still firmly believe in these home-made beauty aids and are bestowed with beautiful, moist, youthful skin.

It is these wonderful women who gave me their secret recipes to be included in this book. I have tried these receipes on myself, my friends and relatives with absolutely astounding results. These beauty aids are safe and pure ingredients—no skin irritating chemicals, no estrogen or hormones in their makeup. They are super-moisturisers and natural lubricants with rich vitamin content in them—everything required to make the skin young, beautiful and alive.

I wrote this books mainly to share these wonderful results with you so that the secrets I discovered could give you the key to a healthy, glowing and beautiful skin —a skin you will be proud of.

ARROONA REEJHSINGHANI

1

Your Skin Story

SKIN IS a part of the body just as the liver, heart and kidneys. When the flow of blood is hindered to the skin for any reason, the skin hardens, thickens and loses its normal appearance. As you grow older in years, the circulation of blood to the skin is lessened and it loses its youthful appearance; its colour changes and wrinkles begin to form on its surface. The speed of ageing starts at 25. It is slow between 30 to 35, fast between 35 to 50 and very quick between 50 to 65. But you can cheat the calendar and preserve your youth by giving your skin regular care and attention both from within and without.

Lack of proper circulation of blood to the skin is mostly due to the lack of proteins, vitamin B and vitamin C. Protein foods supply all the amino-acids essential for keeping your skin youthful. If the proteins and amino-acids are inadequately supplied to the body, the tissues begin to sag causing wrinkles to appear. Like proteins, vitamins are important to the rebuilding of tissues and muscles of the face and body and prevention of wrinkles. Between the cells of the skin is a cementing substance known as collagen which depends upon vitamin C for its elasticity. Always remember that your facial muscles are living elastic tissues and that they can be nourished and built up from inside only with a good and healthy diet. Besides eating a proper beautifying diet there are many other factors which influence the youthful appearance of the face. For instance it is an established fact that the male secretion in the female body makes the skin youthful, brighter, firmer and smoother.

Therefore, many women turn beautiful immedatly after marriage and during the time of pregnancy. Another cause which spoils the skin is the removal of uterus. Its removal heralds in a dry and lustreless and blemished skin. Therefore, if it is very important to your health then only have it removed and that too after consulting a number of specialists and not otherwise. Another enemy of youthful skin is menopause. At this time the body goes through severe physical and hormonal imbalance because the walls of the uterus are papering and drying up. As a result the body stops manufacturing estrogen which is very essential for keeping the skin young. The only remedy for this is to keep the skin moist and supple from outside by the regular use of home-made moisturising creams.

Another main cause of ageing skin is over-exposure of the skin to the sun. This only dries up the skin, accelerates ageing and also darkens it. To slow down this dehydrating process women in tropical countries should drink a lot of water and fruit juces.

Other enemies of youthful skin are regular use of heavy make-up, keeping frequent late nights and consuming too much alcohol. So you see to keep a youthful face you have to take diligent care of your skin. But before you embark upon the programme of looking after your skin you should know the type of skin you have—there are many types of skin. You can broadly classify the types of skin into normal skin, combination skin, greasy skin, dry skin, sallow skin, sensitive skin, chapped skin and withered skin. Now find out into which category your skin falls and give it the treatment as indicated below. Remember it is very important that you use the correct treatment for your type of skin.

Normal Skin

This type of skin has a clear, fine-textured, supple and smooth surface which is neither greasy nor dry. It glows with an inner health which stems from good blood circulation and excellent health. The only care it requires is cleaning it twice a day with a mild baby soap and water. At night, to keep your skin's normal moisture-balance apply a thin film of home-made moisturiser. Any time your skin becomes slightly oily or slightly dry in any area correct these tendencies by following the advice given elsewhere regarding these types of skin.

Combination Skin

Combination skin is a combination of both oily and dry skin. There is a greasy centre panel consisting of nose, forehead and chin and a dry panel consisting of cheeks, mouth and the areas around the eyes. Treat dry areas with home-made cold or moisturing creams and greasy patches with regular application of home-made astringents.

Sensitive Skin

A sensitive skin is a thin or a fine-textured skin. It reacts quickly to both heat and cold; therefore, it sunburns and windburns easily. If you have this type of skin use sun-screen lotions or creams. Wash your face with mild baby soap, rinse thoroughly and pat the skin dry with a soft towel; do not use rough towel. Never use any makeup or perfume without first trying a little of it on the inside of your wrist to see the reaction of your skin to it, for very few items of makeup agree with a sensitive skin. Every night apply home-made moisturising cream on your face before retiring for the night.

Withered Skin

This type of skin has a very rough texture usually full of wrinkles. It is due mainly to over-exposure to extremes of climate such as too much sun or too much cold. To protect yourself from falling a victim to such a skin always use sun-screen lotions or creams whenever you go outdoors for any length of time. Do not use soap; always clean your face with milk cream; it would be a good idea to dispense with soap completely. Use moisturising cream at night. In the morning half an hour before taking bath, take an egg white and mix in one tablespoon of honey and one-fourth teaspoon of carrot juice. Remove with cotton-wool soaked in warm water (to which a dash of soda bicarbonate has been added) after half an hour. This will remove roughness and wrinkles from the skin. Add two tablespoons of olive oil to the water in the tub before taking your bath. Use moisture-laden makeup base in all the seasons and a creamy lipstick.

Chapped Skin

Chapped skin has a rough texture which sometimes

causes the skin to crack. If the cracks develop on your skin then every day at bedtime take the white of an egg, mix in one ground almond and apply on the face. When the skin feels dry, wash off with water and apply home-made nourishing cream. Also avoid the use of soap completely, because soap dissolves the fats from the skin and takes them away from the surface. Instead clean your skin with gram flour made into a paste with milk cream. Half an hour before you take your bath massage yourself either with warm olive, mustard or coconut oil. After bathing blot yourself dry; do not rub vigorously with a bath towel. Apply home-made cold cream every night before retiring. It is a good idea either to use cold or nourishing cream every night after crossing the age of 25 if you want to cherish the youthful loveliness of a flawless complexion. Do not wear woollens or other rough clothing next to your skin because these have been known to aggravate itching and scaling. Always wear white cotton clothes next to your skin—over these you can wear your woollens. If you have developed scales the best remedy is to take a saline bath. Add six pounds of sodium chloride (table salt or rock salt) to 25 gallons of warm water in a tub. Soak in this water for about 15 to 20 minutes twice daily. Blot dry, then massage gently either with almond or olive oil. This simple treatment often brings about a great reduction in chapping and scaling. At the same time it gives considerable relief from itching; but this treatment should only be taken if you are in excellent physical health.

Greasy Skin

Often a chronically oily skin has coarse pores and

pimples and other embarrassing blemishes. If you have an excessively oily skin, take a diet rich in protiens but restricted in sugar, fluids and salt. Also take plenty of leafy green vegetables and fresh fruits. Pork and fried and highly seasoned foods should be avoided. Have your blood brought up to par by the suitable administration of necessary vitamins, iron and similar substances. Besides taking internal care of yourself you should also take equal care of yourself externally. Half an hour before taking your bath apply on your face half teaspoon each of lime and cucumber juice mixed together. If it is excessively oily, mix in a few drops of eau de Cologne. This not only helps keep oiliness away but also helps in refining the pores of the skin by acting as astringent, thereby preventing acne. You must have experienced the problem of your makeup becoming patchy either on the forehead, chin or nose due to excessive oiliness in these areas. To avoid this, apply a little cucumber juice on the excessively oily parts of our face, dry thoroughly and then apply your makeup. But if your whole face turns patchy after makeup is applied on it, then apply equal parts of lime juice and witch-hazel. Dry well before putting on your makeup.

Sallow Skin

Sallow skin has a "No colour look". It is also lustreless and shows lack of vitality that is mainly due to anaemia and lack of vitamins of the 'B' family in your diet. This vitamin, especially vitamin B_1, is very good for curing you of paleness because it keeps the skin well-nourished and rosy by keeping the blood circulation normal. Also active physical exercise will help you because it quickens the blood circulation. Fresh blood and increased oxygen remove all that might dull or blemish the skin.

The 'Hollywood Slant', which is not an exercise but a position, also helps a great deal in combating this trouble. Lie flat on your bed with your feet elevated 12 feet higher than your head. Start with 10 minutes of elevation and gradually work up to 30 minutes. The Cleansing technique depends on whether your skin is dry, oily or normal. If your skin is not sensitive, give yourself a facial once a week to whip up the circulation.

Dry Skin

Dry skin has a parched look caused by its inability to retain moisture. A dry skin is a fine-textured skin and is prone to wrinkles and chapping. It is often a greater problem in cold weather than in warm weather. Use a mild soap for cleansing the skin; follow a bath or a shower with a mild application of baby oil. Massage your face with home-made nourishing cream every night before retiring. Be generous with the cream in the areas surrounding the eyes where tiny lines and crows feet are born. Avoid coming in contact with highly alkaline soaps and detergents like washing sodas and powders which contain highly alkaline and drying ingrediants. Every morning 15 minutes before taking your bath, mix with the egg yolk one teaspoon each of orange juice, olive oil and a few drops each of rose water and lime juice. Another beauty mask is made up of one egg mixed into one teaspoon of honey, half teaspoon of olive oil and a few drops of rose water.

If you can afford it once a week take a milk bath. It will not only nourish and smoothen your skin but at the same time it will also soothe your tense nerves and refresh you. Warm your bath water and put in 250 gram of powdered milk, half tablespoon of almond oil and a few drops of your favourite perfume. Then just lie in it and let your mind wander while the wholesome foam works wonders on your dry skin. If your lips chap, peel or crack then the best remedy is to massage them with a little cream of milk to which a few drops each of rose water and lime juice has been added every night before going to bed. Before applying lipstick, use a soft piece of towelling material for removing rough bits of chaped skin and rub a piece of raw beetroot gently on them. After applying lipstick add a little vaseline to keep your lips soft and pretty.

2

Cosmetics and Dress

In these days of spiralling prices the cosmetic aids sold over the shop counters are beyond the reach of ordinary women. Here are some methods for making your own beauty aids which will not only entail much expenditure in time and money but will also give you the satisfaction of producing genuine stuff. Have you ever envied the lustrous hair of the South Indian women? They owe it to the plain coconut oil.

Make Your Own Cosmetics

Scrape a fresh coconut and grind it to a smooth paste. Squeeze out the milk without using water. Place the juice over a gentle fire and boil it for a few hours till the oil floats to the top, leaving a dark brown residue at the bottom. Remove from fire, cool and strain through a fine cloth. Add any floral essence to this oil and then bottle. This oil is used extensively by the women of Kerala who are famous for their long and lustrous hair.

To make your own shampoo at home scrape a cake of Pears soap very finely, put in a jar and pour in it two cups of boiling water. Set aside to turn into a jelly. This is a plain shampoo. If you want, you can add any essence to it. To make egg shampoo beat an egg with two table-spoons of this jelly and put in essence of choice, put in as much hot water as is required by you and use it.

For making an oil shampoo which is excellent for treating dry hair, put two tablespoons of oil in the soap shreds, then pour in the hot water before setting it aside to jell. Another good shampoo is made by squeezing two limes into the soap shreds. This is an excellent shampoo for treating greasy hair. For very greasy hair mix in half teaspoon of liquid ammonia instead of lime juice,

Nourishing cream keeps the skin soft and supple. Buy six ounces of lanolin and one and a half ounces each of witch-hazel and almond oil. Melt lanolin by placing it in a small bowl. Set the bowl over simmering water. When the lanolin is completly dissolved, remove from heat and beat in witch-hazel and oil and place in air-tight bottle. Nourishing cream is very good for a dry skin.

Make your own bath salts by mixing together 20 teaspoons of epsom salts, six teaspoons of fine table salt and one teaspoon each of boric acid and baking soda. Sprinkle over them a teaspoon of your favourite perfume and you will have a pleasant bubbling bath.

To make your own cold cream buy two ounces of good quality white wax, two ounces rose water and eight ounces almond oil. Melt the wax over top of hot water. Remove from heat and beat in the essence and oil. Cool and bottle.

Make your own eyeliner *kajal*. Fill a clean, sterilised copper, steel or silver *diya* (receptacle) with pure oil or ghee. Make a wick from sterilized cotton and soak it in oil. Light the wick and keep a scrupulously clean copper vessel inverted over the top of the flame about one-third of an inch away from the burning wick. When the oil has been exhausted in the *diya*, remove the inverted vessel and you will find a thick black coating on the vessel. Scrape and powder this well and mix it with a few drops of castor oil to form a thick paste. Place this in an air-tight container. This home-made liner keeps the eyes cool and puts a sparkle in them.

Astringent lotion for tightening the pores. Buy two ounces each of spirit of lavender and eau de Cologne and one ounce of spirit of camphor. Mix together and put in a bottle with tight-fitting stopper. It is excellent for treating a greasy skin.

Here is a recipe for cleansing cream. Three teaspoons of witch-hazel, one teaspoon lemon extract, one teaspoon lanolin, two drops yellow food colouring and six teaspoons of soft shortening. Grind all the ingredients very finely and put in a jar. Store in fridge or in a cool, dry place.

An effective anti-pespirant is made by mixing half ounce of powdered borax, three-fourth ounce of powdered alum with juice of two limes and half litre boiling water. Cool and bottle and use as required.

Do you want smooth arms and legs ? If so, make this depilatory wax. Take 250 gram. of sugar and squeeze in the strained juice of six large limes. Cook the mixture over a gentle fire till it turns light brown and sticky. Remove form fire and mix in one tablespoon of glycerine and store in an airtight bottle. Use when required. If in the hot season this wax turns thin, place it either in the fridge or a bowl of ice till it gets back to the right consistency. If in the cold season it becomes thicker keep the jar for a couple of minutes in hot water.

An inexpensive tooth powder can be made by mixing four teaspoons of powdered chalk with one teaspoon each of powdered sugar and baking soda, flavour with a few drops of oil of peppermint.

For home-made-hand cream mix together to a smooth paste one teaspoon each of soft-shortening, petroleum jelly, almond oil, three teaspoons of lanolin, two teaspoons glycerine and lime juice and half teaspoon of lemon extract. Put in airtight container and store either in the fridge or in a cool and dry place.

You like to smell nice ? Make your own scent. Take some sweet-smelling fresh flowers, a wide-mouthed jar, a little fine salt and olive oil and cotton-wool. Cut the cotton wool in small bits to fit into the jar. Gather the flowers early in the morning when they are fresh. Separate the patals of flowers and sprinkle on them salt, crushing them a little. Soak the cotton-wool pieces nicely. Now place a thick layer of petals at the bottom of the jar and cover with an oil-soaked piece of cotton wool. In this way, go on making layers of petals with cotton-wool in between, till all the petals have been used. Then cover the mouth of the jar tightly. Place the jar in hot sun for 14 days. Remove the lid and squeeze out the perfume from the cotton wool in a clean, sterilised bottle with a tight-fitting lid and use when required. You can make perfume of any flower you like in this way. This home-made deodorant will keep you fresh and fragrant. It also checks perspiration. Mix together three tablespoons each of boric acid powder and salicylic powder in a jar of your favourite talcum powder. Shake up and use.

Tanned by the sun ? Make this whitening cream. Buy one ounce of lanolin, one-fourth ounce almond oil, half ounce each of hydrogen peroxide and glycerine. Melt lanolin over top of hot water. Remove from heat and, while still hot, beat in glycerine and oil. Cool thoroughly and mix in peroxide and a few drops of your favourite essence. Bottle and use when required.

Give Yourself a Facial

A facial is the best treatment you can give yourself. It not only improves thec irculation of blood but also stimulates the muscles of your face. It eases tension and gives a fresh glow to your skin. Tie up your hair, then clean your face with one tablespoon rice flour mixed to a paste with curds, add a pinch of turmeric powder and apply on your face. Rub nicely into the skin, then remove with a piece of cotton-wool soaked in warm water, wash with cold water and then pat dry.

Now take home-made nourishing cream and apply it at the base of the neck, on the sides of the neck, on the chin and araund the mouth, nose and on the cheeks and forehead. Begin by massaging the neck, use your palms from the base of the neck upwards in an upward movement till the chinline. Do this 12 times. Then with all your fingers locked into each other massage once again upwards till the chinline. This stimulates blood circulation and smoothens wrinkles. Now massage the chin in downward movements using the back of your hand. Then beginning at the chinline gently start massaging the face in upward circular movements. As you reach the mouth, do circular movements round the mouth massaging gently with the cushions of your second and third fingers.

Also, massage the lips in the same manner. On the nose, do circular movements with your first finger. Do light tapping with your fingers on your cheeks to increase the circulation of blood in these areas. Gently massage the areas around the eyes in circular motions. Massage the forehead with first finger upwards and outwards in circular motions. This removes tension from the face and induces relaxation. Lastly do the tapping movements all over your face with your fingertips.

Now steam the face. To do this take a medium-sized pan half full of boiling water and make a tent of bath towel over your head. Add herbs or your favourite perfume to make it specially delightful. Steam for about 10 minutes. Pat dry, Now apply a face pack over your face. A face pack deep-cleanses and refines the pores of your skin and improves its colour and texture and gives it a glow or shine. But different types of skin need different types of face packs.

Here are given a number of packs. Choose the one which suits you best:

Greasy skin—Mix together equal quantity of powdered Fuller's earth (*multani mitti*), witch-hazel and rose water to a paste. Blend in a few drops of eau de Cologne.

Dry skin—Mix three tablespoons of oat-meal with olive oil to a paste and mix in two teaspoons of glycerine.

Sallow skin—Beat an egg yolk and mix in half teaspoon of lime juice and half teaspoon of orange-peel-powder.

Dark and dull skin—Mix powdered Fuller's earth to a paste with equal quantities of hydrogen peroxide and witch-hazel.

Patchy skin—Mix together equal quantities of lime juice and olive oil.

Wrinkled skin—Mix together one tablespoon each of honey and egg white along with enough refined flour to a thick paste.

After applying these packs on your face, relax in a darkened room with pads of crushed ice over your eyes in a body slant position. For this position see the chapter on 'Your Skin Story', and read about sallow skin. After about half an hour, wash off, pat dry then dab moisturiser on your skin. Now look at your face in the mirror, it will be tinglingly fresh and glowingly alive. Do not use makeup at all the whole day. Do this once every week if you want to remain young and beautiful always.

Not Skin Deep

Beauty is not skin deep. It has more attributes to it

than the naked eye can see. The attributes that combine to make a real beauty are:

Awareness of others—Aware of not just the exciting few but of everyone and liking all—or if not liking, at least tolerance—the habit of noticing. Others' faults are forgivable or balanced by their equivalent virtues.

Confidence—This takes you right to the centre of things. When you have it you belong everywhere. So what will give you confidence ? Good looks plus good grooming; but that is not all. Confidence means that even when you are faced with an awkward situation, you should not get panicky and you should know how to make the best of it. Be self-assured always.

Good grovming—This should be a part of your regular routine. There is nothing to make you feel so awkward or self-conscious as the knowledge that you have forgotten to wear your deodorant (when you find your escort recoiling from you everytime you go close to him). Good grooming therefore means that you should pay attention to even the smallest item of beauty. You will find this an irksome task in the begining but slowly this will be a habit with you.

Happiness—Happiness is not just cheerfulness or boisterousness, but genuine enjoyement of life. All of us have our bad moments, but real charmers do not cling to them. They know that it is better to be happy than unhappy because happiness attracts people like bees to honey.

Your posture—A bad posture not only effects your personality but also your health. If the body is allowed to sag, the lungs get compressed and the oxygen intake is limited. This also gives rise to improper digestion of food. Therefore, always learn to walk and carry yourself gracefully.

Kindness—It is greatly lacking in this world. A kind word, a helping hand besides giving you inner serenity opens wide the floodgates of good will and fellow feeling.

Alert and knowledgeable mind—For this you need to develop a general interest in what goes on around you by keeping abreast with current news, keeping up with latest fashions and trying to know something about the latest books. Everyone loves an intelligent and lively person; no one cares for a dumb beauty.

Relaxation—Fatigue and emotional disturbances are potential killers of beauty. Chronic worrying brings sleeplessness in its wake, causing wrinkles on your face. Therefore, learn to relax at all times.

Pleasant voice—It is a beauty asset which attracts people. So, cultivate a soft, gentle voice. Tone it with sincerity and polish it to a pleasing pitch and see that your conversation is always pleasant. Be free from ugly gossip.

All the attributes given above are like glowing pearls which will make you into a real beauty.

Good Nutrition

Good nutrition is the starting point on the quest of beauty. When we refer to food we refer to all the nutritive edibles required by the body to keep it fit and healthy. Very often faulty diet gives rise to unpleasant beauty complications like weak and lustreless eyes, blemished complexion, bad teeth, limp hair and other beauty problems. Therefore, if you want to be really beautiful, you should include in your daily diet all the vitamins which help the body to be healthy and attractive, slim and trim. Here are listed all the vitamins which are very essential for keeping yourself beautiful:

Vitamin A—This vitamin corrects and prevents night-blindness and helps the tear ducts to secrete their natural moisture—the best lotion in the world to keep the eyes naturally sparkling and attractive. It also prevents eye-strain and fatigue and keeps them clear and bright, and it is very helpful for hearing properly. A lack of this vitamin can be instrumental in decreasing the hearing capacity. It is also useful for maintaining a clear, bright and youthful complexion.

Carrots are a rich source of this vitamin. Drink a glass of fresh carrot juice daily and see how it puts a sparkle in your eyes and brightens your complexion. Beetroot is another item of food which contains a lot of this vitamin (besides having vitamin C and calcium). This vegetable acts as a laxative and makes the sluggish bowels active. Mustard greens and all types of green leafy vegetables are rich sources of the vitamin A. They are very beneficial for the complexion because they make it blemish-free, smooth and glossy. Amongst these mustard greens helps the complexion to get rid of embarrassing blemishes; spinach has laxative qualities; parsley is an excellent blood-purifier and breath sweetener and the tender leaves of lettuce help the body to relax and get good sleep.

Amongst fruits, apples are a rich source of this vitamin. The malic acid contained in them serves as an antiseptic for teeth, stomach and eyes. Taken last thing after dinner, they help cleanse the teeth. Bananas and papayas are the other sources of this vitamin; they also help prevent constipation. Grapefruit juice, if heated and mixed with honey and taken last thing in the night, helps induce sleep. It also helps people who are hard of hearing.

Vitamin B—This vitamin is very essential for sound hearing. Vitamin B_2 prevents cataracts in the eyes and baldness. The Chinese as a race rarely go bald because they literally live on soya beans, a very rich source of this valuable vitamin. This vitamin prevents early greying of hair and keeps the skin wrinkle-free. Excessively oily and cracked skin can be traced to the lack of this vitamin. Youth and beauty-wise this is an indispensable vitamin. Pigmentation of the skin and ulcers in the mouth can be prevented by this vitamin. It is also helpful for restoring natural colour to the hair. Yeast, a very rich source of this vitamin, is sometimes referred to as anti-grey food. This you can get in the form of tablets and they are known popularly as Brewer's yeast tablets. Increasing baldness, blood-shot and strained eyes can be corrected with this vitamin. Liver, curds and buttermilk are the richest source of this vitamin.

Vitamin C—This is excellent for the eyes and also corrects hearing defects. It gives healthy pink gums and prevents wrinkles. Indian gooseberry or *amla* is the richest source of this vitamin. It prevents tooth decay, brightens the eyes and hair, puts a glow into the complexion and aids digestion. If taken for sufficiently long time it cures almost all the ailments of the digestive tract. Other good sources of this vitamin are liver, tomatoes and oranges. Take a glass of either tomato or orange juice and see your teeth gleam ands hine.

Vitamin D—This is known as the sunshine vitamin because it gives you a sunny smile. It also prevents tooth decay, makes the bones strong, straight and firm and helps to induce sleep. The best source of this vitamin is sunshine. Therefore, always try to relax in the sun for at least two hours daily. Other sources are fish, cod-liver oil, milk, butter and eggs.

Calcium—It is very essential for preventing tooth decay and is very necessary during the growing period—it is during this period that if the blood becomes low in calcium the nerves become irritated and consequently tension sets in. Good sources of calcium are : milk, eggs, cheese, buttermilk, curd and beans.

Iron and Iodine—Iron gives a rosy complexion by preventing anaemia. Liver, apricots, eggs, almonds and soya beans are the rich sources of it. Iodine helps keep the body slim. All the kinds of fish from the sea are the best source of iodine because sea water is the most important source of iodine. It is also found in fresh green vegetables to some extent.

Proteins—The facial skin is made up mainly of proteins. Inadequate intake of proteins causes tissues to sag and the skin to wrinkle. Proteins also assist the natural muscular corset of the abdomen to remain firm and youthful. Its main sources are meat, fish, nuts, poultry, cereals and milk.

Learn to Dress

Do you know what makes a woman stand out in a crowd of pretty faces ? Her clothes. If you are neatly, elegently and suitably dressed for the eccesion you will make heads turn in your direction, but if you are sloppily or unbecomingly dressed, however pretty you may be, no one is going to give you a second look. So, if you wish to belong to that enviable group of well-dressed and sophisticated women, learn to dress with taste and imagination. Wear clothes that suit you, instead of following fashions blindly. Smart women all over the world are never slaves of fashion, they stick to clothes and designs that suit them. Besides helping you in your appearance, the right choice of clothes can work wonders for your figure.

Here are a few helpful hints which will tell you how to camouflage your physical imperfections with clothes. If you are short, you should never wear broad borders or clear horizontal stripes. Broad borders and horizontal stripes will further eat up your height. The best dress for you is the saree for it adds inches to the height. But the saree and the blouse should not be in contrasting colours. They should be of the same shade because this will help carry the eye upwards in an unbroken line giving the illusion of height. Besides being short if you also happen to be plump, you should avoid bright colours and bold designs because they will exaggerate your fullness. In stead, try to wear soft shades because they will make your figure appear slim. If you have a heavy bust, then wear sleeveless and self-coloured blouses and dresses. Wear sarees with contrasting borders, because the border which will run diagonally across your front, will cut the bulk of your figure and give you a slimmer look.

If you have a bulging tummy, avoid wearing buckles, brocches and belts on the centre line. Throw the saree pallav across the shoulder so that the border cuts down the bulge. Accentuate your hair-do. A very beautiful hair-do will draw the eye upwards away from the bulge. If you are tall, learn to be proud of your height. Do not hunch or try to minimise your height by trying to push your neck into your shoulders for this will only spoil you appearance. Wear clothes of contrasting colours and avoid vertical designs. Sarees look beautiful on a tall and slender woman. Wear sarees having broad borders and prints. If you are tall and thin at the same time, then you should wear salwar and kameez, bell-bottoms or pants because they will help to camouflage your height. Avoid tapering heels ; instead wear moderate heels. Absolute flats will make your legs appear longer then they are.

Tall and thin girls sometimes have very thin necks. To camouflage this, wear a delicate odni or a scarf around your neck. This will not only cover the thinness of your neck but will also make you look pretty. Avoid anything delicate in accessories. They are for shorter girls. Carry large purses, wear chunky jewellery and big square wrist watches.

Besides wearing clothes that flatter your figure, learn to choose the right colours for yourself. Before buying any material, drape it over yourself and buy it only if it highlights and adds warmth to your complexion. Never, never choose a colour because it is in fashion or because it suits your friend. Whatever colour you choose, it should always flatter your complexion and not distort your self-colouring. Besides choosing the right shades see that the clothes you wear fit your contours like a glove.

It is much better to have a few dresses which fit you nicely then a wardrobe full of dresses, all poorly designed and put together. If you cannot afford to have your dresses stitched by a good tailor, then try to attend a school of dress-designing and dress-making so that you will be able to make your own clothes economically at home. Keep the clothes you have well-startched, well-pressed and faintly scented. Even the best dress looks ugly if it is unclean, crumpled or smelly.

When you go out, wear clothes which are suitable for the occasion. Pastel shades should be kept for mornings and dark shades should be reserved for the evenings. *Never wear clothes that scream for attention.* A profusion of loud colours used indiscriminately will stamp you as an ill-dressed woman. If you want to add a touch of colour to your outfit, then accentuate it either with an exotic scarf or a piece of costume jewellery. You need not be a beauty queen to appear pleasing and to draw attention to yourself. All you need—to be the centre of attraction—is to be well-dressed. With a good dress sense, you will not only draw attention but also gain confidence and poise at the same time.

3

Hair, Legs, Teeth, Eyes, etc.

To have and to maintain long, lustrous hair one must learn to handle the hair well. If you will give it regular care and attention, you will be amazed with the results —a healthy, shining and beautiful head which will be the envy of every girl you meet on the way.

But before you tackle your hair, you must know to which kind your hair belongs. The hair is roughly of eight kinds: dry hair, greasy hair, curly hair, fine hair, split hair, falling hair, grey hair and sparse hair. Once you know the kind of hair you have and can give yourself the treatment designed for your type of hair, you will be proud of your crowning glory. We deal with each kind of hair below.

Dry hair—Rough, dry hair is mostly the outcome of overuse of perms and dyes and hair sprays or overexposure to oil stealers like the sun, salt, air and sea water. To treat dry hair, take either some warm coconut or olive oil and dab oil along each parting with your fingertips. Continue in this way until the whole scalp has been oiled. Then, massage your head vigorously for five minutes to ensure a thorough spreading of oil.

Two hours later wash your head wiih shikakai. To make your own shikakai at home, take a cup of shikakai seeds and boil them in six cups of water until the seeds soften. Allow to cool, then rub the shikakai between your hands till it turns frothy. Strain through a muslin and use it instead of soap for washing your hair.

Another home remedy for treating dry hair is to soak a big lump of *multani mitti* (Fuller's earth) in a big cup of water. When it softens and becomes a paste add to it two tablespoons of warm cocount oil. Rub it gently into your scalp with your fingertips and later wash off with plenty of water. This treatment will not only cure you of dry hair but at the same time it is very cooling to the eyes and the head and an excellent cleanser.

Even massaging a beaten egg blended with one tablespoon each of lime juice and cocount oil half an hour before going in for your head-bath proves effective in combating a dry scalp. Egg is also good for getting rid of dandruff. Beat white of egg and mix in the juice of sour lime. Rub into your scalp about an hour before you go in for your head-bath. Wash your hair with shikakai and rinse off with warm water to which either a teaspoon of vinegar or lime juice and a few drops of your favourite Cologne has been added. This treatment will surely free your hair from troublesome unsightly scurf. White of an egg, if it is rubbed regularly into the scalp, aids the growth of hair. Egg white, applied well to the scalp, nourishes the hair roots and has cleansing properties as well. Besides on no account should you perm, colour or bleach your hair. Comb hair gently from the roots and smooth over with a soft brush to give them life. Avoid long sessions in the sun without a scarf and always wear a bathing cap when going out to the sea.

Greasy Hair—It is a natural outcome of a greasy skin. If not kept clean, it gives rise to a number of scalp infections. To treat a greasy scalp wash your head with *multani mitti* (Fuller's earth) and *warm* water. (Hot water promotes greasiness). Soak a big lump of *multani mitti* in a glass of water and when it softens, add to it the juice of a big sour lime. Rub it in your scalp and wash off with plenty of water. This not only removes extra oil from the head but proves very cooling to the head specially in the burning hot summer. It also prevents prickly heat and sunstroke. Gram flour too is also a good grease-remover like *multani mitti* and it is used in the same way as *multani mitti.* Another good cooling agent is curd. Take a cup of curd and whisk it till it turns watery. Apply it with your fingertips to your hair roots. Leave on for 15 minutes, then rub your head vigorously with your fingertips till the scalp tingles. Wash off with shikakai and water. Besides being a cooling agent, it darkens the hair and makes it long, lustrous and soft.

Curly hair—This kind of hair is impossible to manage. Yet frequent brushing helps a lot in straightening this type of hair. A very good remedy for straightening this type of hair is to take some warm coconut oil and massage into the scalp, then massage in some water and comb out the curls. Then plait the hair as tightly as possible. Do this every day at bedtime. Another method of straightening the hair is to take the clothes' iron and warm it slightly; then throw your head back on a table and ask someone to straighten out your curls and iron them. Do this once every week. Also set your hair on big rollers to even out the curls.

Fine hair—They are generally limp and tend to cling close to the head. It is alright if they suit your face but they wont if your jaw is full or the features are large. In order to give body to fine hair rub coconut milk into the scalp two hours before you go in for your head-bath. Then wash off with shikakai and water.

Falling hair—The best remedy for falling hair is to wash them with *ritha* nuts. Soak 250 gram *ritha* nuts in four glasses of water in the night. Next morning, boil them for 15 minutes, cool, mash and then strain out the water. Wash with this at least twice a week if you want to get results. Sometimes if you do not check this condition it leads to premature baldness. This is due to a number of reasons, both external and internal. Poor diet is one of the main causes. Other causes are : Hereditary constitutional defects, prolonged illness of certain types (like typhoid) which causes rapid falling of hair due to the presence in the body of certain poisons, blows on the head, pregnancy and menopause, too much exposure to sun, unclean scalp.

A diet rich in iron, iodine and one of the B vitamins, inositol have been instrumental in causing a growth of hair on bald spots. Iodine is responsible for good circulation of blood to the scalp which feeds the minute tube-like depressions known as follicles from which the hair grow. As long as these follicles remain intact and continue to recieve an adequate supply of blood from the body nothing can interfere with the growth of hair. Deficiency of iodine in the body can slow down the blood circulation to the scalp, causing slow growth and falling hair. A lack of iron results in anaemic blood-stream. Some of the vital substances contained in the food are carried by the blood-stream to the scalp. A poor circulation can, therefore, cut off supplies causing deterioration in the conditions of the hair.

Unclean scalp too is greatly responsible for premature baldness. Every healthy hair falls out in four year or less and is replaced by another hair; but unless the scalp is kept scrupulously clean, the new hair may not be able to force its way through. To be sure this does not happen, wash your hair at least twice a week with shikakai and plenty of water. If you wash the hair regularly, your hair will not only turn clean but it will be soft and glossy and free of dandruff.

Dandruff is an infectious condition which arises from

the germs which are normally on the skin but which are more prevalent on a greasy skin. It is usually the outcome of an increase of the secretion from the sweat glands. The best cure for dandruff is lime juice. An hour before you take your hair-bath, rub lime juice to the roots of your hair and then wash it with shikakai. Another good treatment for dandruff is to make partings in your hair and sprinkle oat-meal on it. Leave it for five minutes; then rub the scalp vigorously till it tingles. Remove the corn-meal by thoroughly brushing your hair. After the corn-meal has been removed, press the bristles of the brush on the scalp and push back and forth from side to side for about five minutes. Do this at least twice a week.

Split hair—Trim split ends every month. This prevents the split from reaching up the hair shaft and this also stops the further breakage and damage to the hair. Give your hair a daily message with a little coconut or almond oil. Massage the oil into your scalp with your fingertips until you feel a warm tingling flow of blood in your scalp. Brush the hair for about 10 minutes daily with a brush which should have natural bristles closely set and resilient enough to give a good tug. But it should not be stiff or pointed as it will injure the scalp and split the hair.

Sparse hair—The best treatment for this type of hair is to make partings in your hair and dab in fresh unboiled cow's milk lavishly. Take hair-bath after an hour or so. Do this twice a week. Also give your scalp a good massage with your fingertips for five minutes daily.

Grey hair—It is due to a number of reasons. Greying in many cases is hereditary. Sometimes it is due to emotional disturbances, sudden shock, threat of sudden death or great sorrow. Thyroid gland disturbances can also be responsible through over or under-action. The disease of the pituitary gland is another culprit. Worry, anxiety, mental disturbances and other local skin diseases of the scalp can also cause greying. If Vitamins A and D are deficient in the diet, it gives rise to premature greyness.

However, there are a few things which can be done to help stop or even remove the greying process. In the first place check up your health with the doctor because the general health and all the bodily functions need to be improved. If the thyroid or pituitary gland is disordered, they can be corrected with proper treatment. Warm castor oil and apply it over the whole scalp nicely with your fingertips. Then grip both the sides of your scalp over the ears and massage with your fingers and thumbs for at least 15 minutes. Then go to bed and in the morning have your head-bath. Besides, you can improve the colour of your hair by taking one kilo castor oil and one ounce each of ground coffee and powdered sandlewood. Heat for 20 minutes, strain and keep in a bottle. Massage well with this oil overnight and take your bath in the morning.

Another good remedy for improving the colour of your hair is to take one tablespoon each of *mehandi*, *amla* powder and tea leaves and put in a cup of hot water. Also, mix in one-fourth teaspoon of salt and juice of one lime and half teaspoon of rose water. Leave for five hours, then strain and apply nicely on the hair roots. Leave on for two hours and then rinse with plenty of water. Do this every week and your hair will never turn grey.

If you keep your scalp clean and free of infection, eat the right food, massage daily, there is no reason why your hair should not be alive and shining, long and luxuriant as long as you live.

'Arm' Yourself

Are your arms smooth, supple and shapely or do they tend to be devoid of beauty by being either flabby or plump or too thin or, to crown it all, are they patchy and riddled with superfluous hair? The woman who has neglected her arms should give them extra care and attention before donning the lovely sleeveless dress which is now so much in fashion.

To 'arm' yourself beautifully, you need hardly more then a few minutes daily. Before getting down to improving the texture and the state of your arms, first you must see that they are in shape. If your problem is bulging arms, the best treatment for you is swimming, tennis and badminton because they assist greatly in firming up, the flesh of your arms. On the other hand if your problem is too thin arms, start by using a little psychology on yourself by thinking of your arms as being slender instead of being thin.

Now have a look at your arms. Are they riddled with superfluous hair? If they are, you should get down immediately to remove them. There are many ways of removing these hair and it is up to you decide for yourself which way you would like to adopt to remove them. Have you rough skin on your arms ? Rub salt once a week on the affected portion. Dampen your hand on the affected area and massage a hanful of salt in a rotary movement and then take your bath. A handful of oat-meal soaked in milk for five minutes is another excellent remedy. Message oat-meal on the affected portion, leave on for 15 minutes, than wash off. This not only removes the rough surface skin and makes it soft but also whitens it.

Another good bleaching agent is: mixture of one teaspoon each of tomato, lime juice and milk. After applying, leave on for 15 minutes before washing off. The winter cold works havoc with the oil glands, the glands cannot manufacture body oils quickly enough to counteract the drying effects of the cold wind, to help nature along, massage your arms with top of milk, blended with a few drops each of olive oil and rose wather, five minutes before you go in for your bath. But it is a good idea to always massage a few drops of olive oil into your arms if you want to keep them soft and smooth. If your skin is on the oily side, rub eau de Cologne on them after your bath and then powder them nicely to cut down the over-supply of oil.

The elebows seem to suffer the most from neglect because the thin skin there darkens easily from elbow leaning. So, try to avoid leaning your elbows either on desks or chairs as much as possible. Scrub them every day at bath time with soap and pumice stone. To lighten them cut a lemon into two halves, squeeze out its juice and rest your elbows in the lemon shells for atleast 10 minutes. Do this once every week. And every night before your bedtime massage them nicely with a little top of milk blended with lime or lemon juice.

Your 32 Sparklers

Many people think with growing up, maturing and

growing older a gradual loss of teeth is inevitable. This just isn't true. You should be not only able to smile with your own teeth all your life but you should also see that they are like a string of pearls clean and white. Teeth must be able to cut, tear, crush, grind and shred an enormous variety of food. To do all this work without doing themselves damage, they should be firm.

The roots fit snugly into the sockets in the jawbone but they are not cemented in. Instead, they are cushioned by a thin layer of periadontal membrane and anchored by thousands of tiny fibres which pass from the jaw bone right through the cushioning membrane to the roots. The gums cover and protect this intricate structure and hold the teeth in place. The gums also provide a means for blood to carry oxygen and nourishment to this vital area. When inflammation occurs gums become red and swollen, they bleed and detach from the teeth. This is an indication that the gum tissue has been irritated. Therefore, the area becomes congested with blood which is unable to do its life-giving and disease-fighting job. As the inflammation spreads, first the gum tissue, then the periodontal membrane is eaten away and eventually the roots and the bone-structure supporting the teeth are severely damaged by infection. The teeth get loosened and then they are lost. Therefore, if you have healthy teeth, be good to them: give them regular care and attention.

Here are a few tips on how to keep your teeth healthy and sparkling:

1. Nutritious diet, not age, determines the health of your teeth. Therefore include in your diet calcium, phosphorus and vitamins C and D. These are the four essen-

tial things required for good sound teeth.

2. Clean your mouth with water everytime you eat something because 10 minutes after eating something, acids and decaying agents start attacking the teeth. This is mainly true in the case of sweet and starchy things. Therefore, whenever you consume anything rinse your mouth thoroughly with water.

3. Besides rinsing your mouth regularly, brush your teeth at least twice daily, both morning and night. At the time of brushing, it should be seen that the tooth brush is held under running water for a few seconds to soften out the bristles. Rub the head of the brush not only from corner to corner of the mouth but also up and down in slow circular motions so that it is possible to reach everywhere through the probing bristles.

4. After brushing your teeth message the gums with your fingertips for a few seconds. This encourages the circulation of blood and also prevents the inflammation and bleeding of gums. In case you are already suffering from bleeding gums, mix a little mustard oil with fine salt and massage into your gums a few time daily till you get relief. For pain in the teeth the best treatment is to rub a little oil of cloves into the teeth a few times daily. In case you cannot get this oil, grind a clove to a paste, mix in little water and apply to the affected part.

5. Avoid drinking too many soft drinks because over-indulgence in them causes erosion of tooth structure. Also do not take too many fruit juices (especially, juices of citrus fruits) because they lead to the destruction of local tooth material with harmful effects to the deeper connective tissues.

6. Sometimes due to bad teeth you fall a victim to bad

breath. Make a mouthwash by mixing four teaspoons salt with one teaspoon baking soda, one-fourth teaspoon hydrogen peroxide and a glass of lukewarm water. Gargle with this everytime you have taken your food. Avoid taking onions and garlic and other strong-smelling foods and always keep in your mouth artificial freshners like cardamoms.

7. For sparkling teeth rub your teeth once a week with fine salt and lime juice. This will also help you to get rid of the yellow tint which sometimes occurs on teeth due to neglect. If you want to present a smiling face to the world always keep the few tips given here in your mind.

Show off Your Lovely Legs

Beautiful legs are a great asset especially for girls who like going about in minis and wearing bikinis. Here are some hints to show you how to acquire beautiful legs and feet. For smooth legs 'defuzz' them at least twice a month with a good depilatory. Every morning half an hour before your bath, take one-fourth cup of milk and squeeze in juice of a sour lime and add one teaspoon of olive oil. Mix well and massage it into your legs. At bath time after applying soap to your legs, rub pumice stone on them in a circular motion. This will lessen the growth of hair considerably. Finally, wash your legs and apply baby oil lightly. Do not neglect your feet. Begin with a 10 minute break whenever possible to take pressure off your feet and to allow the blood to circulate more freely.

On specially strenuous days there is nothing like treating yourself to a soothing foot-bath. Dissolve two tablespoons of Epsom salts in a basin of warm water and soak your feet in it for 10 minutes. Dry, then rub baby oil on them. If there is no time for a foot-bath, wash your feet and spray on them chilled eau de Cologne. Feet should be washed often with soap and water. Go barefoot as often as you can to give your feet sun and air and freedom from constriction of shoes. Walking barefoot in the early hours of the morning on dew-covered grass is excellent. This will not only strengthen the muscles of your feet but will also improve your eyesight at the same time.

If your feet pespire profusely (after bathing them with soap and water) dry between the toes and dust freely with salicylic powder. If they become soft and tender, they should be bathed in warm water in which a few grains of alum have been dissolved. Harden tender skin around toes by rubbing with a piece of cotton-wool soaked in eau de Cologne. To keep your feet smooth and supple rub them at bedtime with glycerine. To prevent ugly cracks in winter, rub them with a mixture of lime juice and glycerine every night before bedtime.

If your feet are inclined to swell, put them up whenever you can. Before going to sleep, bathe them in warm water in which a little fine salt has been dissolved and lie down on your bed with your feet raised on a pillow for half an hour. The best way to relax the tired feet is to immerse them in a basin of bearably hot water in which a tablespoon each of salt and turmeric powder have been dissolved. To get instant relief from swollen feet wrap them with napkins dipped in icy water for half an hour. To cure cracks around heels, apply a thick paste made up of turmeric powder and mustard oil every day after taking your bath till you get relief.

If you develop a hard corn nab it while it is fresh. Soak cotton-wool in witch-hazel and apply over the corn; then wear a corn plaster over it. Do this for three days continuously and on the fourth day you will be able to lift the corn without any difficulty. The best remedv for an ingrown toe nail is to cut the nail straight across and gently lift the nail with a clean nail file. Then insert in a small wad of cotton-wool soaked in an antiseptic. Change the cotton-wool twice daily till you get relief.

Athelete's foot is a fungus infection which usually thrives between toes if you neglect to clean them. It causes raw, cracked and itchy skin. It will be cured if you smear the places with alcohol after cleaning and drying them a few times a day. For eczema of the feet the best remedy is juice of *tulsi* leaves. Apply it few times daily to get quick relief. In fact most of the skin ailments of the feet can be cured with the juice of these leaves.

Ill-fitting shoes and socks give rise to most of the foot ailments. Before buying shoes each should be tried and tested to make sure that they are well-fitting and comfortable. Always try shoes on in the afternoon because at this time your feet expand in length as well as in width. Since everyone has one foot larger than the other, try on both the shoes before buying them. Walk around the store to make sure that they are comfortable and fit properly. The prerequisites of good hosiery is that it should absorb moisture and should be non-conductor of heat and at the same time provide adequate protection against heat and cold.

Socks should fit properly providing enough room for

free movement and should not form folds as these rub against the skin and cause blisters. Stretch stockings should be avoided because they constrict the movement of the feet and cause cramps.

Weekly Pedicure—Give your feet a weekly pedicure. You should keep these things handy : nail polish remover, olive oil, hand scissors, nail file, stiff brush, nail polish, orange stick and cotton-wool.

Remove old nail polish with a piece of cotton-wool dipped in nail polish remover or acetone.

Trim your toe nails straight across to prevent painful ingrown toe nails.

File your nails.

Relax your feet for 15 minutes in a basin of bearably hot water to which three tablespoons of salt, juice of half a lime and one teaspoon of rose water has been added.

Apply soap and then scrub well with a stiff brush to remove any dead skin. Wash well in clear water and dry between toes.

Clip away any hang nails and bits of dead skin with the scissors.

Wrap cotton-wool round an orange stick and soak in warm olive oil.

Gently work this round the base of the nails pressing the cuticle back and removing dead cuticles.

Soak the feet again in warm, soapy water. Wash well and dry thoroughly.

Before applying polish, place small swabs of cotton between each toe and then apply polish. Allow the first coat of polish to dry thoroughly and then apply the second coat.

Your Own Special Eye Care

The most neglected part of the body is the eyes, and yet it is the eyes on which the whole beauty of the face depends. But we punish them by giving them little or no rest and we strave them continually of food which they need to keep themselves strong, bright and clear. In spite of treating them so inconsiderately they serve us faithfully. If from now on you are even casually 'decent' with them, they will respond eagerly. Here are a few tips telling you how to take care of them :

1. Feed vitamin A, B and C to the eyes because it is mainly these three vitamins on which the health and beauty of your eyes depends. Vitamin A prevents night-blindness and fatigue and puts a sparkle into your eyes, while vitamins B and C prevent eye-strain and cataracts. Therefore, these three vitamins along with other vitamins should be fed regularly to the eyes if you want them to serve you faithfully throughout your life.

2. Reading in strong or dim light, dazzling or flickering light, reading small or bad print, or reading in a stooping posture or lying down or going frequently to the movies, or reading in moving cars and trains should be scrupulously avoided as all this cause, severe eye-strain.

3. To soothe, clear, brighten and refresh tired eyes bathe them daily in chilled pure rose water.

4. To relax tired eyes, rub your whole face with ice, then dip two cotton-wool pads in iced water and place them on your closed eyelids. Lie down in a darkened room for 10 minutes and relax by having your feet up against the wall. By having your feet higher than your head, the blood moves towards the heart and refreshes the whole system including the eyes.

5. Take at least eight hours' sleep in the night. In the morning and evening, splash your eyes hard with tap water to get wide-awake feeling, tone the eye-muscles and to clean and remove impurities from within.

6. Never put any lotions, eye drops, fruit juices and oils in the eyes without consulting a very competent eye specialist because eyes are very delicate organs of your body and if these things do not agree with them they will harm them beyond repair—causing even total blindness.

7. Any complaint of the eyes should be immediately treated by the best eye specialist in your town or city. If you make no effort to correct the condition, it might cost you your sight.

8. If your doctor recommends spectacles get yourself the best that money can buy. Well-fitted, good looking ones help you to feel and look years younger because they remove tension and strain from your eyes. Wear them only when you absolutely need them. Give the muscles of your eyes every chance to relax, which they cannot do with spectacles on. Even if you cannot do without them, take them off from time to time during the day, close your eyes, cup your palms over them shutting out all light and forget the world for at least 5 minutes.

9. To get rid of deep dark circles from under the eyes take eight hours' sleep every night. Take a diet rich in fruits and vegetables and avoid reading late at night or going through long hours of work or any work requiring close visual concentration like sewing, reading and writing. Alternate hot and cold compresses under your eyes for 10 minutes, then apply a teaspoon or almond oil mixed with half teaspoon of lime juice on the dark surfaces

every night before going to bed. Every morning, after washing your face gently apply equal mixture of tomato and lime juice and then take your bath after half an hour or so. Every week bleach the areas with hydrogen and ammonia mixture. Lastly see that you get plenty of fresh air and exercise daily by going for long brisk walks both in the morning and evening.

Beauty at Your Finger-tips

Lovely hands tell the most flattering things about you. They give you confidence and are a symbol of femininity. Pretty hands are not easy to acquire (with the daily domestic chores we all have to do) but with a little care and attention you can, if you like, make them beautiful. The use of detergents, the ill effects of successive cold and hot water, the manual work involved in cookery will in the long run dissolve all the natural oils secreted by the skin, making wrinkles to appear on the surface of the skin and giving an old and aged appearance to the hands.

Therefore, whenever you do any manual work, wear rubber gloves lined with cotton. They are cheap and easily available at all good chemists' shops. Every night before going to your bed, take one teaspoon top-of-milk and mix in one ground almond and a few drops each of lime juice, glycerine and rose water. Massage the mixture into your hands. Next morning, apply a little gram flour on your hands and wash them nicely. This treatment will not only make your hands soft and smooth but at the same time they will make them fairer. To remove stains from your hands either rub them with raw potato slices or lime slices. For stubborn stains try soaking them for five minutes in equal quantities of either vinegar and water or lime juice and water.

The best cure for cracked and rough hands is to apply on them regularly camphor cream. To make this cream take one cup of sesame seed oil and mix in one ounce each of pure wax and camphor. Heat the mixture till all the ingredients dissolve and then store in a clean bottle or a jar. Wash and dry hands, then apply regularly at bedtime. In the cold season the hands turn red and swollen, the best cure for this is to soak them for 10 minutes in salt water. Dry with a soft towel and massage into them one tablespoon of top-of-milk mixed with a few drops of glycerine.

Hands are apt to be stained while cutting vegetables. The best way to stop this is to always grease your hands with a little oil before cutting. To remove any strong smell from your hands take a tablespoon of gram flour. Mix in a few drops of lime juice and enough water to make it into a paste. Apply on the hands nicely, leave for five minutes. Then wash nicely with water. With good hands you should also aim at having attractive nails. To improve brittle and splitting nails caused by lack of calcium, take gelatin. Every morning take a glass of milk or fruit juice and mix in two tablespoons of powdered gelatin. After two months you will find definite improvement in your condition. In addition apply some white iodine with a stick wrapped in cotton-wool along the cuticles and under the tips of the nails daily to strenghten them. Every week give your nails an oil bath. Take a little warm olive oil and put it in two squeezed out lime halves. Dig your nails in the halves and let them remain thus for about five minutes before washing them with soap and water.

A weekly manicure is a must if you want your nails to set off the loveliness of your hands. Before starting your manicure assemble together the following items : a packet of emery boards (because they are less liable to damage the nails), cotton-wool, a bottle of cuticle remover, a bottle of acetone for removing old nail polish, a bottle of your favourite shade of nail polish. Place all these items on a tray as well as a bowl of warm soapy water and a small hand towel. Then :

1. Remove any old polish with acetone.

2. Shape your nails with the emery board working from the outer corner of the nail to the centre.

3. Soak hands in soapy water and dry with the towel.

4. Massage the cuticle cream into your hands. Wrap the tip of a toothpick with a little cotton-wool and soak it in cuticle remover, gently work this round the base of the nails pressing the cuticle back and removing dead cuticle as you go.

6. Now apply the base coat. The easiest way is to make a dab in the centre of the nail, outline a half-moon with one stroke of the brush then fill in the whole nail. Wipe tip of each newly polished nail carefully with a piece of cotton-wool to leave a hairline free of polish so that it would not chip easily.

7. Allow the first coat to dry thoroughly before applying the second coat. When the second coat is completely dry apply one tablespoon top-of-milk blended with a few drops of lime juice and your favourite Cologne on your hands and wrists and then wash off with soap and water after a few minutes. The best all-purpose nail polish is one of the pale pink shades, but it goes without saying

that whatever shade you choose, it should not clash with your lipstick.

4

Beauty and the Seasons

To look beautiful in all the climes and seasons is mostly a matter of experience and technique. Given a few tips, a woman can ever be beautiful, anytime and anywhere. India, a vast country, has varying seasons and climates. So, the sooner an Indian woman learns to adjust to the changing seasons—to keep beauty as also to enhance it—the better.

Beauty and the Monsoon

Here are a few beauty tips specially for the monsoon which will keep you cheerful and glowing right through the wet season. First of all, you should learn to wear the right type of clothes. The clothes you choose to wear should not soak up water easily and even if they do they should dry up quickly without losing shape. Put away all your crisp, cool cottons and silks because they not only soak up water avidly but become limp when they dry and lose their crease and shape completely. Synthetics like nylon and terylene are ideal for this season because they are crease-resisting, dry up fast and regain their original shape when dry. Wear vivid, vibrant colours—glowing turquoise, rich green, deep orange—to beat the grey rainy days. Buy a bright raincoat and a matching umbrella to go with it.

Wear rubber or plastic shoes during this season to prevent your feet from getting wet. Following exposure to rain, remove wet shoes immediately on reaching home. Wash your feet thoroughly in warm, soapy water, then rinse in clear water and dry up. Massage them vigorously for five minutes and change to dry shoes. Never wear wet shoes again without drying them thoroughly, otherwise you will be vulnerable to a host of diseases ranging from common cold to pneumonia. Always keep an extra pair of shoes at your place of work or in your bag so that you can change into them if your shoes get wet. A good way of drying wet shoes quickly is to stuff them lightly with crumpled newspaper, then dry them in the kitchen, away from direct heat of the fire. It is a good idea to message glycerine on your feet every night before going to bed. This will help to keep your feet soft, smooth and free from skin ailments.

During this season you should avoid using foundation and face cream when going out because rain will wash it off leaving stained lines on the face. Confine yourself to using lipstick, rouge, eyebrow pencil and powder. Use lipstick of a deep, vibrant shade and apply a dash, a lipgloss, to put a glow in your lips. Use rouge sparingly. Blend it carefully into the skin; see that it is a glow of colour and not an ugly red spot. Pencil your brows in a series of fine lines and never in the form of a curved thick line with one swing of the pencil. The final effect should be a natural looking arch. Finish your makeup with light puff of powder.

The watchword for hair-do is simplicity. Avoid back-combing and lacquer, intricate buns, curk and waves, because the humidity in air will make your hair limp and ugly within next to no time. Either make a single plait or a plain bun. Wet hair like wet feet gives rise to a number of diseases. Therefore, to dry hair quickly, buy a portable hair dryer. This will not only dry your hair in a few minutes and give you a well-groomed look even on a very wet day but it will also save the 'doctor's bills'.

Use an egg mask once a week. Take white of an egg and mix with one teaspoon each of honey and lime juice. Apply over your face and leave for one hour. Then wash off with warm water and splash on cold water. If your face has natural tendency towards dryness it will be more obvious during this season. Take the yolk of an egg and mix it with a teaspoon of cream of milk and a few drops of rose water. Apply on the face and neck, leave on for 15 minutes and then wash off.

Cool and Composed during Summer

The kiss of summer bestows nature's shining secret to your face as long as you do not let it dry your skin and cause those tiny summer wrinkles to appear. Try some of the suggestions given below to revive and to sustain the natural beauty of your complexion and to add that cool, clear appearance, which is the main asset of a summer complexion. During the hot summer months your complexion needs extra care at night in order to counteract the drying effects of the sun and the wind during the day. Particularly, if you are above 25 you should regularly use a moisturising cream at bedtime. Apply this cream daily in the night if you want to cherish the youthful loveliness of a flawless complexion.

To make your own moisturising cream take four almonds and soak them in enough milk to cover them. Let them remain thus for a whole night, next morning peel and grind them to a smooth paste. Now mix in two tablespoons of milk cream and a few drops of essence of rose. Store in a bottle and keep it in the fridge.

As the tempreture rises in the hot months, extra cleaning is necessary for those of you who have greasy complexion. Bathe your face four to five times daily with clear water and a good soap suited to your complexion. This will help cleanse the openings of grease glands and loosen excess secretion. Rinse off every trace of soap with plenty of hot, then cold water. Cold water constricts the pores and minimises the entrance of dust and dirt into the oil glands. Now splash an astringent lotion on the face. In a bowl of chilled water squeeze in a juice of a sour lime. Pat dry. Remember to cleanse the skin thoroughly with milk cream blended into a thin paste with gram flour. Steam the face once every week in order to open clogged pores.

Another big problem of summer is excessive pespiration and body odour. Excessive pespiration usually occurs on the palms, soles, under the breast, forehead and scalp. It is often accompanied by offensive body odour which is largely due to the decomposition of sweat and contamination with micro-organisms. Under unclean circumstances, micro-organisms flourish giving rise to unsightly boils. Therefore, if you suffer from foul-smelling pespiration, you should pay special attention to your personal cleanliness. You should take bath twice daily with soap and plenty of water. Certain areas of the body (where pespiration is excessive) should be dusted liberally with boric powder mixed with an equal quantity of a good-scented talcum powder. If your feet pespire profusely then use salicylic powder on them or you can soak them for 15 minutes in a dilute solution of potassium permanganate in order to prevent infection and minimise body odour. Refrain from wearing nylon or woollen socks. Wear cotton socks and shoes which have no rubber soles on them. To check pespiration of the hands wash them well, dry them, then rub them with a few drops of witch-hazel.

Infants and toddlers should be bathed in the afternoon in water to which a few drops of Cologne have been added. Dust their bodies libearlly with equal quantity of scented powder and boric powder. For top-to-toe freshness pay proper attention to your hair. It is important that you should wash your hair at least twice a week. Freshen your hair in between by sprinkling some eau de Cologne before setting them. Revive tired eyes by wrapping crushed pieces of ice in a piece of cloth and applying it to closed eyelids. Then relax for 10 minutes in a dark room. You can use cucumber slices instead of ice cubes.

Ensure that feeling of freshness by keeping yourself and all your personal belongings, scrupulously clean. Your sarees, dresses and other clothes should be starched and well-pressed for a neat appearance. Keep pads soaked in cologne between your clothes and they will exude a lovely fragrance. When ironing your clothes, place a pad of cotton soaked in either Cologne rose water or your favourite perfume by your side and run the pad on your clothes before ironing. Your pleasantly fragant clothes will make you feel cool and garden-fresh. Do away with all your nylons, georgettes and heavy silks and bring out the soft wispy *chanderies*, cool violes, crisp organdies and light cotton dresses in the softest of shades. Avoid wearing too many accessories.

During this season your makeup should be reduced to the minimum and the accent should be on naturalness. Avoid using foundation creams and lotions of any sort because heat may cause them 'running down' your face. Use a lipstick of pastel shade and use rouge sparingly. Finish your makeup with a light puff of powder.

Be extravagant with flowers. Use plenty of them in your hair. You can also tuck a few flowers of *mogra* in your bra for their heavenly smell. Spray on your favourite perfume and now if you go out you will feel as pleasantly fresh and cool as though you were atop a hill station in the summer season.

Complexion Care in Winter

Winter is dreaded by many because usually it brings a challenge to every complexion, but you can look your best if you take a few precautions. During the winter months your complexion needs extra care and attention because the oil glands just below the surface of the skin become relatively inactive and produce less moisture than usual. This and the increased dryness of the skin due to the drying effects of the sun and the wind are responsible for causing the tiny wrinkles and giving rise to various skin ailments like scaling, itching, chapping and eczema.

The best way, however, to counteract these ailments is to dispense with the use of soap completely, because it has been known to have a marked de-greasing action on the skin. Instead, clean your face with milk cream or top-of-milk blended with a few drops of lime juice and a pinch of turmeric powder. Excessive use of cosmetics, hair dyes and sprays, too many hot baths and perfumes also make the hair dry. Every night before going to bed, take one tablespoon of milk cream and mix in a few drops each of glycerine, olive oil and rose water. Mix well and apply over your entire face, neck and hands. Leave overnight; in the morning wipe off gently with a tissue paper, then bathe the skin in warm water until it begins to feel warm and also rinse for the same length of time in cold water. Pat dry with a soft towel.

Also, massage your body well with olive or coconut oil blended with a few drops of rose water 10 minutes before your bath to make your skin soft and glowing. If dryness has resulted in scaling, take foods rich in vitamin A, because this vitamin is stored in the fat just below the surface of the skin counteracting any tendency towards dryness and roughness. In case the scaling is quite severe, also take this vitamin in the form of tablets but as this vitamin sometimes produces toxic effects in the body if taken indiscriminately, it should only be taken under medical supervision.

Another common skin ailment in winter is eczema. Initially the surface of the skin becomes red but later it turns dry, rough and scaly. Here are two effective remedies for this ailment. Grind a walnut to a paste, squeeze out its oil and apply on the affected parts a few times daily. In case this does not give relief, try this remedy. Take a dry coconut and hold it with a pair of tongs over a burning flame. When its skin turns completely black and while it is still burning, place it on a tin-plate and cover it immediately with a small vessel. Remove it after a few seconds and you will find a layer of oil on the vessel. Rub this on the affected parts twice daily and within a week you will find definite relief in your condition.

Itching too is a common complaint during this weather. Take a tablespoon of sandlewood oil and mix in an equal quantity of coconut oil. Apply on the itching parts of the body a couple of times daily until you get relief. The juice of *tulsi* leaves is also equally effective.

Another type of itching which is very severe is known as winter's itch. This is usually due to the excessive dryness of the skin. It is also due to wearing too many woollen garments, too many hot baths, too little sun, lack of sweating, too much use of soaps and scent and dietary deficiencies. Arms and legs are commonly affected by it. To minimise winter's itch, every day an hour before taking your bath take two tablespoons each of curd and olive oil and mix in a few drops of essence of rose. Mix well and apply on the body an hour before you take your bath. Abstain from wearing woollens next to the body. Reduce hot baths and the use of the soap to the minimum. Take vitamin A in the form of tablets and expose yourself to the sun for at least an hour daily. It automatically disappears in the warm weather because perspiration caused by the heat helps to keep the skin soft and moist.

If the skin on the soles of your feet becomes hard and

cracked, rub the soles at bath time with soapy water and pumice stone. After bathing be sure to dry the feet well especially between the toes to prevent cracking. Massage them well with olive or coconut oil to keep the skin soft and smooth and to help the circulation of blood. After exposure to cold, take a foot bath using warm water and soap. Wipe dry, massage them vigorously for five minutes and then wear woollen socks. This is very important to prevent chilblains.

If your lips happen to chap, peel or crack, here is an effective remedy. Take a rose flower and grind the petals to a paste. Mix in a little cream of milk and apply it generously on the lips before going to bed in the night. This will help keep the lips soft and pretty. Dry, itchy skin around the mouth is a common complaint during winter. Vitamin B tablets will help in this case.

To protect your hands from rash and chaping wear a pair of rubber gloves when doing household chores. Every night before going to bed take an equal quantity of lime juice, glycerine, rose water and Cologne and apply nicely on the hands and after you finish your household chores rub glycerine and sugar on them for a couple of minutes and then wash off. This will help keep them soft and smooth.

Winter plays havoc with the hair, making it dry, brittle and dull. To bring a healthy shine to your hair, take some warm coconut oil, make partings along the hair and dab it along each parting with your finger-tips. Continue in this way till the whole scalp has been oiled, then wrap hot towels over the head to keep the scalp as warm as possible. After half an hour when the scalp has absorbed oil, wash the hair with shikakai and water.

Hair can never be completely clean and shiny until it is rinsed thoroughly—it should squeak at your touch.

Use a moisturized foundation to protect your skin against the harsh effects of the cold weather. Touch up your lips with warm, creamy colours. Pale lipsticks will make you look pale and sickly in this weather. Add lip-gloss or a little vaseline to keep your lips soft and pretty.

Also follow a healthy diet scheme to enable your body to fight against the many ills of winter and to put an attractive bloom in your cheeks.

5

Beauty and Age

EACH AGE-GROUP has its own problems and Beauty has to contend with them. Toddlers and children have to be handled in a way that they learn personal hygiene and beauty care. Similarly, teenage girls, young women and middle-aged women should understand the nature of the demands of their age-groups and do beauty-care accordingly.

Growing up with Beauty

If you have given birth to a baby girl, start looking

after her beauty from right now if you want her to be a beauty queen when she grows up, for the foundation of beauty is laid in childhood. Heredity gives a child the colour of her skin, the basic bone structure and the texture of her hair, but the rest depends upon careful nurturing, diet and exercise.

To a very great extent good looks depend upon the type of food a child is given to eat. If a child is given an adequate diet it will build up her bones, muscles and blood and give her sound teeth, smooth and firm skin and bright hair and glowing eyes. An adequate diet is made up of a great variety of foods from which the body obtains the necessary elements for its growth. The essential elements are vitamin A which aids the vision, helps the teeth form and keeps the skin firm and smooth. It is found in fresh green and yellow vegetables, butter and eggs. Vitamin B which is very essential for a child's growth is found in whole wheat, mutton, pulses and lentils and milk. Vitamin C which is very essential for healthy gums and teeth is found in citrus fruits and tomatoes. Vitamin D which helps keep the bones strong, straight and firm is found in sardines and fish liver oil. Calcium which builds and maintains strong bones, teeth and nails is found in plenty in potatoes, whole milk, buttermilk and cheese. Proteins which build and repair the body are found in all kinds of fish, mutton, poultry, cereals and nuts.

All the foods listed above are very important for general health and for giving energy. Therefore, you should see that your child is given all the above items of food in her diet. But see that you do not give your child too many sweet and fatty foods because these are not only bad for her figure but will lead later to poor digestion and spotty complexion. However, if your child happens to be very fond of sweets, them give her home-made sweets made with honey instead of sagar. Instead of soft drinks, give her juices of fresh vegetables and fruits. Besides giving your child good food see that she has some form of exercise daily. Dancing is the best form of exercise for every girl, because later on it will not only give her poise but will also make her body graceful and slim. Besides dancing, swimming and swinging are the other forms of exercise which every child should take. Swimming will provide her with a shapely bust-line later on and swinging will make her grow tall.

Babies and small children can also have their skin problems. If the child has an occasional pimple then be very careful because such children easily fall victims to acne in later life. Cut down on greasy and starchy foods and keep her skin scrupulously clean with a mild baby soap and water. Juice of mint leaves if applied twice a weak on the face every night before going to bed till after passing adolescence will help greatly in combating acne and other embarrassing blemishes.

If your baby is born with dark fuzzy hair on her face, arms and legs, take a little rose water and cream of milk and mix into a smooth and thick paste. Apply the paste all over her and let it turn a little dry, rub the paste very gently for a few minutes on her body and then give her, her bath. This will not only help to remove the superfluous hair but will also improve her complexion. Besides applying the paste, dilute a little lime juice in equal quantities of rose water and apply on the parts on which she has hair, for if some of the hair remain in spite of applying the gram flour paste, they will be golden and not black because lime juice is a very effective hair bleacher.

Children have lovely soft hair which only needs cleaning regularly with a mild baby shampoo. However, if your baby's hair is too fine, then rub fresh cow's milk in to her hair roots 15 minutes before giving her head-bath. If they happen to be too curly and unmanageable, then after giving her head-bath, apply a little oil on her hair and plait them. Do this regularly every alternate day for a few months if you want results. If her scalp happens to be dry, then massage it gently with pure glycerine and let it remain for 10 minutes before washing her head.

Children usually get lice and nits in their hair in spite of keeping them clean because lice come through contact with other children who might not be as clean as your child. Lice give rise to many skin diseases. Therefore, as soon as you find that your child has lice in her head take one small packet of camphur and dissolve it in four tablespoons of pure coconut oil. Make partings along her hair and dab the oil into each parting with your finger-tips. When the whole scalp is oiled, tie the head with a piece of muslin and let it remain so the wholo night. Next morning, give her, her head-bath. Do this treatment at least once a month till she is in school if you want her head to be free of lice in spite of being in contact with other children. To remove nits, wet the hair thoroughly with hot vinegar and comb with a fine-toothed comb.

Never keep your child's hair greasy for children never look their best with greasy hair. Always apply oil to their heads before shampooing their hair and never afterwards. Trim her hair every two months so that the split ends are removed and the nourishment in the hair goes entirely to the hair shaft. Do not braid her hair too tightly and never tie it up in a tight pony tail for later on due to this, the hair start falling and breaking. Children should be encouraged to play or run around bare feet for sometime daily, as this exercises the muscles of the feet and makes them strong.

When a child is just learning to walk, shoes should be very soft and flexible. Too tight shoes and socks can easily distort young feet. And do not forget her teeth because they are the main assent of a beautiful face. Teach your child to brush her teeth after every meal up and down on gums and teeth and not sideways. Make her wash her mouth thoroughly with water after eating sweets because long after a sweet has disappeared into the stomach, its sugar lingers on in the mouth in contact with the teeth, eating away into its enamel. Therefore it is very essential that she should be made to rinse her mouth with water because water washes away these concentrated sugars from the mouth. If she has crooked teath, take her to a dental surgeon. He will use braces in her teeth to make them straight. By giving your child necessary care and attention at a young age she will not only grow up to be a very beautiful damsel, but she will also have confidence and poise—the basic qualities for charm.

If so far you have not paid much attention to your child's looks, start from now on so that she leads a happy and healthy life later on.

Beauty for the Teenagers

The developing young body of a teenager leads to a variety of problems. Some of the most common problems being underactive glands, resulting in various skin troubles like acne and open pores and overweight and underweight problems. If you are overweight (or if this is your tendency), you have to pull out any sweet tooth that you might have and do it immediately. Instead of rich and creamy desserts and sugar-laden drinks, take more milk and eat more nourishing vegetables and fruits. Also, adequate (not giant) servings of meat, fish, poultry and eggs are essential to your health and good figure. But if you are underweight, you must choose foods with high protein and vitamin content. Don't skip meals and don't try to substitute them with quick snacks at odd intervals. That is one of the worst eating habits you can have, which will not help you to round out those angular corners.

Besides taking a proper diet, sleep for at least eight hours daily because the skin cells can only renew themselves while you are asleep. Exercise in fresh air. Go for long brisk walks both in the morning and in the evening. During growing years your skin will be getting coarser and the pores will get accumulated with secretion leading to embarrassing bumps and blemishes. To escape this and to keep the skin taut, moist and glowing, keep your skin clean by cleaning it thrice a day 'religiously'. Steam your face at least twice a week. Then, apply a mask made up of two tablespoons dried orange peel powder made into a paste with milk and little rose water. This mask not only cleans the skin but also purifies the pores of your skin so that they function in the way nature intended them to.

Take good care of your hair because this will pay you rich dividends in later years. Brush it nicely both morning and night and if you have reason to think that your hair is falling unduly or looking dull give it the treatment prescribed earlier. And if you have fallen a victim to acne, follow the advice given elsewhere. As for makeup use compact on the face and the palest shade of lipstick available in the market. Apply lipgloss on it if you like. Instead of mascara, brush a little castor oil on your lashes; this will not only give them a wider look but will at the same time encourage their growth. And as for the nailpolish use palest of the pink shades.

Be a Beautiful Bride

Every bride-to-be wants to look her loveliest on her wedding day, the most exciting day of her life. To look bewitching on that day, you should start beautifying yourself a day in advance.

Look at your arms and legs. Have they unwanted growth of hair ? If you have hair there, then 'defuzz' them for a well-groomed look. Give yourself a pedicure and manicure and then bleach your face with one tablespoon of hydrogen peroxide mixed with a few drops of liquid ammonia. Follow with a facial and then go in for your head-bath. On the big day, before applying your makeup, *you should first take a bath.* This is an absolute must if you want to face your hubby fresh and fragrant.

Take your bath with a fragrant soap and water in which you should put a few drops of perfume of your choice. If you use warm water, then finish off with a cold shower, because cold water closes the pores of the skin and minimises the entrance of dirt and dust into them and therefore the skin does not fall a prey to embarrassing blemishes. Now take a towel and quickly rid your body of surplus water. Follow this with very vigorous rubbing with a coarse towel until you are fairly glowing. This way you exercise the skin and improve the circulation of blood. As you dry your hands and feet, press back the cuticles. When you are dry, use underarm deodorant and powder yourself with a fragrant powder.

Now you should leave the bathroom and start with your makeup. Before applying your makeup, you should keep in your mind that you should look as natural as possible. Your husband wants to see you the way he is used to seeing you. He wants you to look lovely, sweet and natural and not some painted doll. Use foundations first. You should use a pinkish tone to brighten up your complexion; then apply rouge, which will lend a gentle blush to your face.

Eye makeup should be applied deftly. Remember that your eyes are your most expressive features. Therefore, accentuate them nicely. Use an eyeliner which will help elongate your eyes and make them appear larger. Mascara will help your lashes appear longer and thicker. Arch your brows slightly following your natural line. See that the colours of your lipstck matches your saree.

Apply lipgloss over your lipstick for a scintillating effect. Make a simple hair style. Do not dress your hair in some fantastic new style. Fantastic hair do will make you look anything but lovely. Brush your hair vigorously to give it body and shine and then make a simple hair style. Decorate your hair with fresh fragrant flowers.

Apply perfume—do not forget to apply it on the palms of your hands. Wear your clothes and jewellery and step out of your room to meet and bewitch him—your man.

Beauty after Twentyfive

A woman having a perfect, petal-smooth and rosy complexion is the envy of all women. Wherever she goes, heads turn in her direction in admiration. Such a complexion cannot be acquired without an effort. It has to be cultivated slowly and gradually by nurturing it carefully from within and without. Up to the age of 25 the skin is naturally supple, glowing and alive, but it is after the mid-twenties that the skin slowly starts losing its fresh and youthful appearance and acquiring a parched look. This is because the cells deep within the skin layers are no longer able to retain their moisture and the beauty of the skin mainly depends upon the moisture contained in the cells. The skin which cannot retain its moisture turns dry, rough, dull and wrinkled. Therefore in order to avoid looking prematurely old, you should try to observe a basic skin-care routine after you pass your mid-twenties so that the cells in your skin can retain maximum moisture and your skin remains firm, moist and young right up to old age.

Some people believe erroneously that moisturising creams and lotions alone will keep the moisture level of the skin in perfect balance. No surface addition of moisture and no man-made lubricant will help you unless you look after the inner life of your skin where beauty and youth really begin. Therefore, if you want to stimulate your cells to activity for a new look and the feel of youth, feed it regularly with a diet rich in proteins and vitamins B and C. Also, take at least six glasses of water every day, one glass of carrot juiue and one pint of either milk or buttermilk. Besides looking after the inner life of your skin, you should also look after its outer life.

It is a good idea to use home-made moisturizing cream regulary after the age of 25 onwards, because this cream helps keep the skin soft, dewy and alive. But before applying any cream, remove all traces of make-up with home-made cleansing cream. Foundation cream is not soluble in water and does not come off even with soap. Therefore, a cleansing cream is a must for removing every trace of makeup and grime sooty and coaly dirt. To make the cream take one tablespoon of gram flour and mix to a paste with cream of milk. Stir in a few drops of lime juice and a pinch of turmeric powder. Mix well and apply it with your finger-tips over your face and neck. Leave it on for a few mintes and then rub your face vigorously with your hands. The paste will go on falling as you rub. Remove the clinging paste with hot water, splash on cold water. Blot dry and then apply this home-made cream on the face and neck. Blanch and grind four almonds, one walnut, a couple each of peanuts and charoli to a very smooth paste. Mix in four tablespoons of cream of milk, two melted. tablespoons of cucumber juice and one table-spoon each of honey and rose water. Mix well and store in a small bottle. Massage it on the face and neck in circular upward movements firmly and gently.

This cleansing cream should not be just patted on the skin but it should be rubbed hard into the skin so that the oils it contains are picked up by the glands. But be careful with the areas around the eyes. Pat the cream lightly using the middle finger-tip under and around the eyes. Leave the cream on for half an hour and then remove with tissue paper what the skin has not absorbed. This cream will not only give you a normal skin which is neither dry nor greasy but at the same time it will give your skin a natural glow, the look of health and feel of youth.

After you cross 25 use only moisture-laden foundation creams because they not only protect a dry skin and help maintain a normal skin but also protect the skin from wind, sun, cold and dust.

Use a special moisturising pomade stick on your lips before applying your lipstick and apply over it a little lipgloss to keep them soft and pretty.

If you take regular care of your skin after you have passed your mid-twenties by feeding it with a sensible diet and using moisture-laden creams, the cells of your skin will be supplied with ample moisture to keep it supple, soft and wrinkle-free. Your skin will have a smooth surface that is neither oily nor dry with a glow of health that stems from good blood circulation, regular care, regular attention and excellent general health.

Beauty after the Forties

There are very few women who keep on looking beautiful even after crossing the age of forty; but these women have cultivated their beauty slowly and gradually through the years and they age gracefully and carry their years as lightly and gaily as flowers in a buttonhole. In later years, a slim and trim figure adds as much to the look of youth as a youthful skin. To keep your skin slim, eat a fully balanced diet, because after you cross the age of 40 there is a marked decrease in the functional activity of the body. The process of digestion slows down, therefore the fats and the carbohydrate content of the diet should be reduced. Fried foods and dishes of carbohydrates should be avoided.

Overweight persons need to be all the more cautious of their calorie intake because they are more prone to old age diseases than their slimmer brethren and sisters. Therefore, take food rich in vitamins and minerals and avoid sugary, starchy and fried foods like plague. Eat plenty of fresh fruits and vegetables and drink at least two cups of milk daily.

With the onset of age the hair becomes grey, but do not pull these grey hair out. Every time you pull out a grey hair, you sow the seed for another few because the root at the base of the hair folicle secretes an infectious serum, which covers a tiny pinpoint of healthy hair surrounding the white hair and these in turn will go white within next to no time. If you feel you must get rid of your grey hair then cut it close to the root with scissors.

Keep your hair well-brushed, well-nourished, well-groomed and styled at all times. This is the time when your skin needs an ample amount of grease to counteract the natural dryness of your skin. Every night apply home-made moisturising cream to your face and in the morning before you take your bath, rub on your face and neck home-made cold cream. Pay particular attention to the corners of your mouth, areas around the eyes and neck which are more prone to wrinkling than the other areas of the skin. Give yourself a facial twice a week with a mask for dry skin to whip up circulation.

Do not wear clothes and makeup used by the teen-agers; wear clothes suitable for your age, which will give you dignity and good bearing. Wear light makeup and simple jewellery. Besides develop a lively interest in all things and have a sense of humour at all times which will give your face a nice tender look and not a frowning, cross look (which adds years to the face). Go for long brisk walks and do not look back more than you can help at your green years, for remember that every age has its own charm. Moreover, after 40 you have much more mature and dignified look than before. Therefore keep your shoulders back, hold your head high and above all, keep the corners of your mouth up.

Beauty-Care for the Working Woman

A career woman is a very busy woman. She has not only to go to office and handle a lot of exacting chores but she has also to look after the household after her responsibilities at the desk are over. This leaves her with little time to look after herself and yet she needs to look neat and attractive in her place of work. What you require is to take one day off every week and *reserve it for beautifying yourself*. Make it Sunday when usually everyone has a holiday. This day should belong exclusively to you. Rest, relax and beautify yourself and see how the next day you will not only look more beautiful and attractive but be lighter and brighter both in body and spirit. This one day beauty-care is not only meant to beautify you but it is also health-giving and prolongs your youthfulness. On this day be as 'lazy' as possible, stay in bed as long as you like and stay off the telephone because talking takes as much energy as working.

Take a light diet on this day to give your over-worked digestive system a rest. Here is a sample of the Sunday diet.

Breakfast

One glass orange juice
Cornflakes with milk
Tea or coffee.

Mid-morning

One cup skimmed milk with 1 biscuit. (You can substitute milk for tea or coffee.)

Lunch

Steamed chicken or fish
One roti
One green or yellow vegetable
One salad of raw vegetables
Fruit of choice.

Mid-afternoon

Tea, coffee, milk or soft drink with 1 biscuit.

Dinner

Soup
Mutton stew
Bread
Fruit.

Bedtime

One cup skimmed milk with honey.

After taking your breakfast, rest for a while and then go in for your bath. Lock yourself in and get to work. Start with chores like 'defuzzing' your legs or arms, dealing with suerpfluous hair on the face, washing and setting your hair and doing your nails. All these chores need to be done regularly for a well-groomed look.

Now take your bath. Fill the bathtub with lukewarm water and put in a few drops of your favourite essence. Then, lie back in the tub and try to keep your mind blank—think of absolutely nothing for 10 minutes or try to dwell upon happy things. Let your arms and legs float in the water, splash them around a little and let the ripples in the bath water float over you. Get out of the bath and pat yourself dry and give yourself a facial.

After all this, you should emerge from the bathroom, both refreshed and invigorated. Now have your lunch and go to bed. *Do not talk, do not gossip, do not work*, for this day is for you and for the next six days you will be for others—what a relaxed, beautiful and changed person you will be !

As regards the skin, clean your face both morning and night because, as you are out in the open for long periods, your skin takes on more dust and grime than the women who stay at home.

However tired you may be after a late night, do not hop into your bed without removing every trace of your make-up otherwise your pores will get clogged and your skin will become sick. Every night before going to bed give your skin a little nourishment by rubbing in a little cream of milk blended with lime juice and a pinch of turmeric powder. Use only a dusting of powder, a soft shade of lipstick and a touch of rouge for the office. And always carry your makeup kit with you to 'do' yourself up before leaving for your home.

Also pay greatest attention to your personal cleanliness so that you will not only feel fragrant but also fresh and lively the whole day through. So use a little bath essence, toilet water and dusting powder and also use deoderant regularly whether you think you need it or not.

Beauty during Pregnancy

Pregnancy is nine months long and with proper preparation many of the ordinary discomforts and beauty problems of pregnancy can be avoided, giving a feeling of well-being and great satisfaction. The inevitable result of bearing a child is that the infant draws upon the mother's reserves, thus making her undernourished, sickly and pale. To avoid this eat a nourishing diet. If the daily supplies of food are sufficient, the bones, teeth, hair, eyes, skin and the mother's other reserves will not be drawn upon and the infant will be properly supported on 'income' and not on mother's 'capital'.

A pregnant woman should daily take: at least four cups of milk; two or more fruits, one of which should be citrus; two or more vegetables, one of which should be deep green or yellow; one dish of potatoes;. one or more eggs; 250 gram or more of either meat, fish or poultry; three to four servings of either whole grain or bread; four tablespoons of butter; one multivitamin tablet; two calcium tablets and one fish liver oil capsule.

The food mentioned above will provide for the maintenance of the mother's body with enough extra to take care of the tissue growth of the infant, enough calcium and vitamin D for basic development and enough iron to prevent anaemia in the mother and to supply all the needs of the infant.

Constipation is a very common problem during pregnancy and, if not checked, it gives rise to a number of embarrassing skin blemishes. To cure it drink at least eight glasses of water every day. Besides, include laxative fruits like figs, prunes and beetroots in your daily diet.

As the abdomen becomes larger, the skin stretches. Fibres of the connective tissue immediately underlying the skin separate and give rise to white stretch marks. To avoid these, it is always wise to massage the abdomen and the breasts regularly with oil from the first month of pregnancy right to the last and even after delivery—for a few months at least. On no account scratch the abdomen and the breasts, because this will leave scratch marks for ever afterwards on the skin. If you feel very itchy, gently—very gently—rub the skin with your hands.

If you are planning on breast feeding your baby, you should begin preparing your nipples from the sixth month onwards. Once every day, draw out each nipple by gently pressing your thumb and index finger down on either side of the nipples and gently rolling the nipple out. After your nipple stands out, massage it well with little olive oil. Nursing will not cause your breasts to become flabby, if you wear well-fitting brassiers. Buy yourself a few maternity dresses, which today come in many attractive designs and shapes. Do not forget that a large 'percentage' of attractiveness is accounted for by good grooming and good posture.

The clothes should be comfortable and well-fitting with allowances for future expansion. Also discard high-heeled shoes and wear comfortable low-heeled flat shoes.

Towards the later months many women develop varicose veins. Varicose veins is a disease in which the veins become very enlarged and protrude out of the skin. Varicose veins mostly develop in the legs. The women who develop this condition are the ones whose occupation requires standing or sitting for long periods.

It is wise that during pregnancy, you do as much of your work as possible in a sitting position with your feet propped up. When you have to be on your feet, it is better to move around than to stand still. If you develop this condition, wear plastic stockings before you get up from your bed. Report your condition immediately to your doctor. Besides, you should lie down at least once every day for at least one hour in a body-slant position. (See 'Sallow Skin' in Chapter 1) for this position.

Sometimes swelling of legs, ankles, feet, fingers—and face too—may appear during the last months. The cause of swelling is the retention of water in the tissue spaces of the body; a high intake of salt favours the retention of water, which is why you should eliminate or use very little salt in your diet and reduce the intake of liquids.

The pressure of the body on the large blood vessels in the later months may give rise occasionally to bouts of light-headedness and sometimes fainting. If this occurs, you will feel better if you lie down for a few minutes. Also increase your intake of iron.

Sometimes your sleep maybe interrupted by hard muscular cramps in the calves of your legs. Massage the cramped area vigorously and apply hot water bottle or heating pad to the area.

Heartburn and flatulence are the other common disturbances of pregnancy. Heartburn is a kind of burning feeling which is noted at the lower end of the breast bone–therefore, the name Heartburn. To prevent this eat smaller meals at regular intervals rather then the bigger ones. To prevent flatulence or the formation of gas in the body, eat light and nourishing foods rather than rich and heavy foods.

Proper care of the skin and hair (as described in the previous pages) is specially important during pregnancy. A daily bath with a mild fragrant soap is a must. Clean your skin both morning and night with milk cream to which a little lime juice and turmeric powder has been added. Every morning before you go in for your bath take a teaspoon of curd and mix in a few drops each of almond oil and essence of rose. Rub it well into the skin and remove with cotton-wool. This will soothe and feed the skin.

For the night make this skin-food: to four tablespoons of cream of milk add one tablespoon each of almond oil, cucumber juice, honey, rose water and lime juice. Mix well and put in a small jar and store either in the fridge or a cool, dry place. Apply every night before going to bed. Remove in the morning with a piece of cotton-wool, then splash on cold water. This will put a bloom on your cheeks and sparkle in your complexion.

Wear minimum of makeup. If you have a tendency to develop rashes it will be exaggerated during pregnancy. Sometimes pigmentation of the skin takes place or the formation of small areas in which the minute skin veins become prominent. There is no remedy for these ailments but they disappear soon after pregnancy. You should give up all our social engagements and lead a very moderate life. Your motto should be—Early to Bed and

Early to Rise. Good sleep, fresh air, regular skin-care, exercise coupled with right diet should give you health, strength and beauty throughout the time you are 'expecting.'

6

Makeup

THERE ARE no ugly women in this world: there are only two kinds of women—the beautiful and the plain. The former are the women who have realised the beauty potiential latent within themselves while the latter are those who have not realised it yet. But it is the duty of every woman to try and look beautiful at all times.

The Magic of Makeup

The plainest girl too can stand out in a sea of beautiful faces with a few clever makeup tricks. Makeup is a gift of modern times which gives every woman the opportunity to present her best face to the world at all times. But the secret of makeup is to underdo it; it should be subtle, natural and suited to the personality of the woman who wears it.

Begin your makeup with foundation because it is the

basis of all makeup. As the term indicates it is the basis upon which your makeup is built. The way the foundation looks on the skin depends upon how it is applied and blended. As a general rule apply the foundation sparingly and on a clean skin only. Cleanse the skin with top of milk blended with a few drops of lime juice. Then, wash off with soap and plenty of water. Pat it dry with a clean soft napkin. If your skin happens to be on the oily side, rub a piece of tomato on the face after washing it with soap and water and leave on for five minutes. Again wash with water and pat it dry. Let the skin rest for a few minutes and then put on the foundation.

Select a foundation cream which is of the colour of your skin or a shade darker than it. If your skin happens to be on the oily side, you will do well with a liquid foundation and a dry skin does better with a creamy foundation. If you have a lovely natural skin, a mild application of liquid foundation will help to enhance your natural loveliness. With the help of your fingertips, apply a little on the forehead, ears, cheek-bones, nose and under the chin, front and back of the neck. Blend thoroughly with upward and outward strokes over the entire face under the jawline back to ears, over and around the eyelids and mouth. Cover all the visible areas of the face and the neck. A few extra seconds of blending and gentle rubbing will give the desired even finish.

After the foundation comes the face powder. It follows the initial application of the foundation, serving as a coverup and lending that matt (lustreless) finish to the foundation-cream. Select a powder in your skin tone colour or it should be one shade lighter than your skin tone. It is important that both the shade of the powder and the foundation should be of a matching tone.

If your skin happens to be pale then intensify it with a slightly perky note. If it is swarthy, use a pink tan tone. If it is sallow, aim for a slightly cream rose effect. Take a pad of cotton-wool and press the powder gently on your face and neck till the skin becomes smooth and matty in appearance. Allow the powder to set for a few minutes and then gently dust off excess powder with a powder brush. Brush in downward strokes as this helps to flatten tiny facial hair and gives a smooth finish.

Then comes the rouge. It puts a glow on your cheeks and imparts a bright and healthy look to your face. However, the rouge will not look right until it is very skilfully blended into the skin so that it should not be obvious that it is being used at all. It should be applied so sparingly that it should only give a faint glow to the complexion that would otherwise look pale. Always go in for a light coloured cream rouge because very dark and purplish shades add years to the face. Take a little rouge on the tips of your two middle fingers and pat lightly on the cheekbone where the natural colour is supposed to be. Then, blend the colour well in so that no hard lines are visible.

After the rouge comes the eye makeup. Right type of eye makeup has the most dramatic impact on your whole face. But before you start make sure that you have all the essentials at hand—tweezers, eye brow pencil, eye shadow, mascara and eyeliner. Take a look at your eyebrows. Are they uneven, too short or too long ? Is there a straggly growth of hair on the bridge of your nose. They give an unattractive frowning look to the face. The only answer to this is to reshape them. Before starting to reshape them, keep in mind that beautiful eyebrows should curve up away from the nose and tail off gracefully at the temple end. Also remember that the most beautiful eyes are so spread that in the distance between them another eye can be placed. Take the sting out of the tweezing by bathing the brows in warm water. Dab them dry; apply a little olive oil mixed with a few drops of eau de Cologne on them before starting the tweezing. Now take your tweezers and holding the surrounding area taut, grip the hair close to the roots and give a sharp tug in the direction the hair grows.

To prevent the skin from bulging after the plucking has been done, wrap an ice cube in a piece of cloth and gently massage the area. Plucking should be done every alternate day for a constant well-groomed look. If your brows are scanty or too light, use an eyebrow pencil to accentuate them. The pencil should be black as black brows predominate in our country. Brush your brows with a clean mascara brush into a smooth arch and define them slightly with light feathery touches with the pencil. The pencil must be used to tint the actual hair of the brow and not the flesh in between. The final effect should be a natural looking arch. A well-shaped dark brow on the other hand may require no pencilling but just a neat brushing with either a little vaseline or cream. In case you have very sparse brows then encourage their growth by applying a little castor oil blended with a little raw cow's milk.

After the eyebrow pencil comes the eyeshadow. It gives brilliance, depth and life to the eyes. The safest shade to use is soft blue. However, there are no rigid colour rules.

It can match or contrast with the eye colour. It is often more effective and dramatic when it harmonises with the colour of your dress. Before applying the shadows use both foundation and powder over the eyelids. Eye shadow should be blended on the upper lid. Close one eye and then apply a narrow strip of shadow with your finger-tips next to the upper eyelashes from inner to outer corner of the eye, blend it with your finger-tips up and out over the eyelid but see that it is darkest near the lid. You can also use two shades of shadow one next to the lashes and the other over the rest of the lid. The shadow nearest to the lashes should be of a deeper shade than the one used on the rest of the lid. The use of a deeper shade close to the lids gives the eyes extra depth and definition.

Now comes the eyeliner. A soft line drawn next to the upper lashline with eyeliner makes the eyes larger and brighter. It is available in three forms—liquid, cake and pencil. Liquid liner is preferable because it is waterproof and does not smudge or pull the skin around the lid. To line upper lashes with index finger hold outer corner of eyelid taut. Then draw a soft line with eyeliner from inner to outer corner as close as possible to the lashes. Taper off the line before it reaches the inner corner of the eye and also taper it off where it finishes at the outer corner of the eyes or a little beyond. To line lower lid, hold the lower lid down with the index finger and away from the eye and then draw a faint line on the narrow ridge above the lower lashes. This will appear light and subtle but will make the eyes appear larger and brighter.

Now comes the turn of the mascara. Mascara is a must for the starry-eyed look, for it makes the lashes appear longer and thicker. First brush the lashes downwards to remove surplus powder then upwards. Mascara goes on better under a fan. The lashes do not gum together due to the air. Always apply it with a clean brush. Cover the brush with a light coating of mascara and stroke it from the roots to the tips of the lashes slanting the strokes slightly towards the outer corners of the eyes and coaxing as many lashes as possible beyond the corners to create a wide-eyed look. Maximum glamour is achived if you take the mascara right upto the eyeliner so that the dark colour of mascara meets the dark colour of the eyeliner to create the glamorous look. Let the first coat dry completely; then apply the second coat, for two thin coats look more natural than one thick coat. Dry again; then separate the lashes with a dry brush.

Use a cotton-tipped stick dipped in warm water to remove any smudges from the lids. For the stunning glamour-girl-look after the mascara is completely dry, take a little gold or silver eyeshadow on your finger-tip and stroke the ends of the upper lashes from below. This proves very effective for the late night parties. If your lashes are thin or sparse you can try false eyelashes. But it requires a great deal of patience, skill and time to put them on. First put on eyeliner and mascara on your own lashes to curve them, then apply glue thinly on the base of the lashes. Do the following to make the lash strip supple and easier to fit. Hold strip with both ends, curve it into an N-shape, then raise and lower alternate ends in a continuous sinuous movement till the glue dries up a bit. Then, place a mirror on the table, look down into it, drop lashes onto the lid—use end of liner brush to press strip into place.

Women who wear glasses can also make the most of eye makeup. Rather then mask out the eyes, glasses draw attention to them and so you can do with the maximum use of eye makeup. Use eye shadow because it flatters the eyes behind the lens and helps to absorb the glare. Use an exotic shade in the evenings to give your eyes an extra impact. Use mascara in moderation on the upper lid but there should be just a suspicion of it on the lower lid.

Now use the lipstick. Learn to master the technique of using lipstick by learning to use the lipstick brush, if you want your lips to took beautiful and inviting. Stroke the brush forwards and backwards across the lipstick and as you do this coax the bristles into a wedge shape with a fine edge. Use this keen edge to outline your lips, Steady your hand by placing the elbow on a firm surface, let one hand support the chin while the other handles the brush.

Fashion the upper lip first with the lips slightly apart. Draw the outline from the corners to the centre of the lip; then sharply outline the cupid's bow. Use the side of the brush on the lower lip working at one-half of the lip at a time. When the outline is clearly established, fill in generously with colour. Allow to set for a few minutes, then blot on a tissue paper, apply lipstick again. Give them a dewy look with a touch of vaseline, cold cream or lip gloss. Lipstick colour should complement the complexion tone and harmonise with the colour of your clothes. Brown, yellow and emerald green colours look nice with a red lipstick with some yellowy tone. Pastel colours look becoming with soft pinks. Blacks and whites call for something bright and dashing whereas for mauves and lilacs cyclamen lipstick will do. Wear pastel shades of lipstick in the morning and for the evening use deeper shades to minimise the effect of the electric lights.

And now, finally, comes the perfume. Perfume should be used as a finishing touch to good grooming. Perfume helps a woman to appear alluring and attractive always. Therefore, make it a habit of using it always so that it becomes a part of your personality. From the wide range of perfumes available in the market, select the one which is most suitable to you. A perfume must establish a trademark for your personality—something that will evoke memories of you even when you are miles away.

When selecting a perfume, do not just sniff at the bottle; dab some on your wrist and leave for a while till the fragrance settles then let your nose be the judge. Do not buy a perfume just because it smells good on a friend because it's reaction depends mainly upon the chemistry of your skin. Once you have bought for yourself the right perfume, use it to the best advantage. Use it on the throat, earlobes, behied the ears, wrists, nape of the neck, temples, inside the crooks of the elbows and chest. Perfume applied on these pulse spots stays alive because of the warmth of the skin at these spots, the body heat releases the fragrance and you will be enveloped in an exciting, mysterious, alluring and utterly irresistible fragrance.

An economical use of perfume is to soak a piece of white flannel in it and tuck it either in your bra or at waist where the warmth of yonr skin sends the fragrance out as you move. Always carry a phial of perfume in your bag with your lipstick and compact. Thus when you renew your makeup, you can also renew your charm.

Never apply perfume on your clothes because it can stain them and never apply it after wearing your pearls, silver or artificial jewellery, because it will harm them beyond repair. Always apply perfume, leave on for 5 minutes and then wear your jewellery and *zari* clothes. On an oily skin the perfume clings longer. Therefore, use it sparingly but if your skin is on the dry side add an extra dash for good measure. Finally, never make the mistake of applying the perfume just before leaving your house as thus the scent will vanish quickly in open air. Apply at least 20 minutes in advance to give it time to settle down. If you cannot afford to include expensive perfume in your wardrobe, use a good Cologne. This must be used more lavishly to give you a delicate lingering fragrance and garden fresh feeling.

Art of Becoming Beautiful

Makeup is a gift which, if used correctly, can transform even a plain looking woman into a breathtaking beauty. Makeup, if expertly applied, corrects defects and emphasises the best features. Correct makeup tricks camouflage facial defects and heighten or bring out natural beauty. To determine as to which features should be subdued and which should be emphasised, study the front and the profile of your face carefully in the mirror and decide for yourself where corrective makeup is necessary. Here are a few hints for you to follow:

Chin

Double chin—Apply normal foundation colour, then pat a lighter shade on the appropriate part of chin and blend it right round the chin.

Receding chin—Apply normal foundation colour, then place a thin line of lighter foundation in the natural hollow just below the lower lip. Blend well, powder with a shade lighter than the one applied to the rest of the face.

Prominent chin—Use a darker foundation on the chin and powder with a corresponding shade of powdr.

Pointed chin—Pat a lighter foundation round the edge of the chin and blend into the foundation colouer. Powder with a shade lighter than the one which is applied on the rest of the face.

Lips

Thick lips—They can be made to look thinner by painting within the natural lipline and covering the remaining area with foundation cream.

Thin lips—If the lips are too thin, the upper lips can be extended a little above the natural lipline but care must be taken to see that the extended portion follows the natural curve of the lips. The lower lip should be full and well-shaped by extending the lipline a little below the natural lipline of the lower lip.

Drooping lips—To perfect this condition, straighten curves with fuller lines to the corners.

Small mouth—Extend the corners of both the lips.

Eyes

Close set eyes—Apply eye shadow to the upper eyelids, blending the shadow upwards and outwards towards the outer corner of the eyes.

Continue to blend until the shadow is considerable fainter in the area of the nose and the eye and somewhat darker at the outer corner. Then with the help of the brow pencil, draw a line a third away from the inner corner of the eye and extend the line beyond the outer corner. Blend the line so that like the shadow it is faint at the inner corners and darker at the outer corners. Increase the distance between the eyebrows by tweezing to make them appear wider apart.

Deep-set eyes—Use a lighter foundation colour immediately above the socket area of the upper eyelids and blend with the foundation colour. Do not use eyeshadow as the sunken effect will increase instead of decreasing.

Drooping eyes—They can be given a lift by tilting the eyeline upwards and outwards before it reaches the outer corner of the upper lid. The shadow should be winged upwards avoiding the area at the outer corner of the eyes.

Round eyes—Make them appear longer by extending eyeshadow beyond the outer corner of the eyes.

Bulging eyes—Use a dark shadow and blend it carefully over the prominent part of the upper lids carrying it lightly to the line of the brows.

Small eyes—They can look larger by using two kinds of shadow. Use brown shadow on the lip creases after applying 'biege' to the lids.

Face

Long narrow face—Blend the rouge back from the cheekbones to the hairline in an almost straight line. This creates a horizontal effect which adds width to the face. Do not bring rouge close to the nose as then the widening effect will be lost.

Square face—This looks more oval if the rouge is shaded in long triangle towards the cheekbones.

Hollow cheeks—They appear fuller and rounder if the rouge is blended above the hollows instead of being blended in the hollows. This application neutralises the natural shadows in the hollows and makes them appear rounder and fuller.

Oval face—Dot rouge on the height of cheekbones under centre of the eyes. Blend up and out until the edges disappear.

Round widish face—Keep rouge fairly close to the nose, blend up at sharp verticrla angle to the outer corner of the eye to give illusion of length.

Ears

Large ears—Apply deeper foundation to the ears. This will make them appear less conspicuous. Wear large earrings which clamp on your earlobes and cover them.

Forehead

Bulging forehead—Use a deeper foundation just below the temples over the eyelids and on the upper part of the nose. This will give an illusion of fullness to the rest of face and minimise the bulge.

Low forehead—Apply a lighter foundation on the forehead so that the space between the eyebrows and hairline appears broader.

Nose

Broad nose—Use a darker foundation to slim a broad nose, blending from nostrils upwards towards the bridge of the nose. Then powder the nose with one shade darker than the one applied to the rest of the face.

Long nose—Apply normal foundation first, apply darker foundation to the base of the nose and blend upwards and over the tip of the nose.

Thin nose—Apply normal foundation from the nostrils to the bridge of the nose in up and down movements. Powder the face with one shade lighter than the one applied to the rest of the face.

Flat nose—After applying normal foundation colour, apply a lighter foundation colour straight down the centre of the nose from just above the bridge to a point just below the tip of the nose. Powder with your normal powder.

Neck

Short and thick neck—Use a darker foundation on the neck than the one used on the face to make the neck appear thinner.

Long thin neck—Use a lighter foundation on the neck than the one used on the face. This will create an illusion of fullness and the neck will not appear so thin.

Dark shadows under the eyes—Disguise dark shadows by using a pale foundation under yonr normal makeup.

Freckles

To tone down freckles and to give yourself a creamier look, use a foundation slightly less pink than your natural colouring. Then powder with your normal face powder.

Age lines

Age lines and crevices can be concealed by applying the foundation cream evenly with an outward circular movement over your skin.

Scars and Pimples

If they are visible, blot them off with a colour darker than applied to the rest of the face. Dab the area with this colour blending the edges in with the rest of the foundation. Then powder with your normal powder.

Tired look

A very light touch of rouge in the centre of your forehead will go a long way in banishing a tired look from your face.

Different Categories of Makeup

Makeup generally falls into three major categories: morning makeup, evening makeup and gala evening makeup. Besides these three types of makeup, different types of skins require different types of makeup. Here we describe the different types of makeup.

Morning makeup—Keep morning makeup as light as possible because the harsh rays of the sun pitilessly point out all the makeup defects which go unnoticed in the mellow light of the evening. Avoid using foundation or face cream of any type, but if you must apply it, do it very sparsely and near an open window and not in a closed room under artificial lights. Lightly apply rouge, put on soft shade of lipstick, puff on some powder, add eyeliner and a thin coating of mascara.

Evening makeup—You can use foundation but use it lightly and blend it well into the skin. Besides, you can include rouge, dashing shade of lipstick, powder, eyeliner, mascara and eyeshadow but in a muted tone.

Gala evening makeup—Gala cvening makeup or night makeup is a heavier type of makeup. You can use all the makeup tricks without looking out of place or you can even add a touch of glamour to your appearance by sprinkling silver dust on your hair and applying silver eyeshadow to your eyelashes.

Now comes the makeup for various types of skins.

Dry skin—Select moisture-laden foundation cream and a creamy type of rouge and shimmering lipstick and lipgloss to go with it. Use creamy eyeshadow and liquid eyeliner.

Greasy skin—Buy an astringent lotion and put it on before makeup to cut down oily skin shine. Use a greaseless medicated foundation that gives an even matt (lustreless) finish to your skin. Puff the powder on in a blotting motion using a fresh piece of cotton each time.

Sallow skin—Use a moisture-laden foundation in a warmer tone than your complexion. plexion. Follow with a compressed rouge coloured powder to give a fresh glow to your face and use warm shades of lipstick and eyeshadow.

Pimply skin—For a pimply skin avoid using face creams and all types of skin foods, lubricants and face creams. Use only medicated antiseptic foundation and face powder which help to heal as well as flatter the complexion. However, more emphasis should be put on the use of lipstick and eye makeup in order to draw attention to your eyes and mouth so that your pimpled skin is less noticeable.

Makeup when you are sick—You have probably noticed that your skin has a tendency to be blotchy whenever you suffer from cold or any other sickness. Over a film of foundation cream dust on pure white talcum powder. This will impart on all-over radiance to your skin. Apply creamy rouge and a vibrant shade of lipstick because this will add colour to your face and give you a healthier look.

7

Skin Ailments

THERE ARE many a skin ailment from which almost every person suffers at one time or another. There are certain habits, ways of living, ageing process and climate, etc. which cause these ailments. Most of these ailments can be cured very easily. Some of them occur at a particular age.

Acne—An affliction of growing years, acne is often the cause of acute mental anguish and embarrassment to the teenager. But it can be successfully treated at home. Here are a few home remedies with easy-to-follow advice. Whatever you do, never attempt to treat acne by picking or squeezing the eruptions. This will not only spread it but will also cause untold damage to the skin tissue. Tiny black-capped eruptions are called blackheads which can be dislodged by enlarging the pores with steaming facials and gentle pressure.

Begin this facial by cleaning the face thoroughly with

cleansing cream and then take a medium-sized pan, half full of boiling water. Make a tent of a bath towel over your head, steam your face for 10 minutes. Once again clean your face with the cream. This will remove surface-skin blackheads. After the steam bath heat the white of an egg to a stiff froth. Add a few drops of rose water and apply it on your face. Leave it on until your face feels stiff and wash it off with water. This egg mask closes and tones the pores and checks oiliness. Another effective mask is Fuller's mask. Mix Fuller's earth to a smooth paste with rose water and apply on the face. When dry, wash off with water. Wipe dry. Then rub with a rough napkin to dislodge the blackheads.

For deep-seated blackheads take seven cups of hot water and mix in two tablespoons of boric powder. Dip a clean napkin in this water and swathe your face in it. When it turns cold, repeat the procedure. Do this for about 10 minutes. This will help remove the grease and soften the blackheads. After this heating process squeeze out the blackheads with the help of an expressor, which is an instrument made specially for this purpose. It has a small spear-like point at one end and a cup-shaped spoon bearing a small central hole at the other end. It is best to prick the apex of the blackheads with the sharp point before using pressure. If numerous large and closely grouped superficial blackheads are present, you can remove them by taking a piece of ordinary adhesive plaster. Heat the plaster and apply it firmly over the affected area. Leave it on for 24 hours and then pull it off with a sharp tug. This method, if properly used, is very effective for removing blackheads. This procedure may be repeated but it should not be used on sensitive or very hairy areas. After removing them dab dilute alcohol or some mild disinfectant on the skin.

Whiteheads are tiny cysts which are formed due to the improper elimination of oil secreted from the grease glands. They have the appearance of hard white spots and they appear on any part of the body, but they are most commonly seen on the areas around the face, especially nose, cheeks, temples and forehead. A whitehead can be best removed by steaming the face for five minutes over a bowl of boiling water. When the whiteheads in the pores have been softened, prick the apex with a clean sterilised needle and gently, very gently press it out with your fingers.

Never let the fingernail press the skin and never squeeze the skin. This can cause scars and broken veins. Another very effective method of removing whiteheads is to rub them regularly with a mixture of mild soap solution and table salt, then wash off with cold water. After a few rubbings the whiteheads can be removed by gently pressing them out.

Pimples

If blackheads and whiteheads are not checked and treated immediately, they harden and decompose into pimples. Pimples are small red boils, sometimes coming to a head and sometimes not. There usually is some pus inside and sometimes blackheads are present in the pores.

There are several remedies for treating this condition which are noted down here and you should make use of the one which suits you best. Mix sandlewood with rose water to a paste or mix Fuller's earth with rose water to a paste and apply on the face half an hour before you take your bath. Do not use soap or creams or lotions on the face until you are cured of this condition. Another effective remedy is to mix one tablespoon of gram flour with half teaspoon of powdered dry *neem* leaves, pinch of turmeric powder and two teaspoons of milk to a thick paste. Apply it in the same way as sandalwood mask.

An effective remedy for the pimple (that has suddenly appeared on the face) consists of applying of starch made into a paste with water at night before retiring. Next morning, the pimple vanishes as though by magic.

The spots which result from pimples, blackheads and whiteheads can be removed by grinding an almond to a paste and mixing with one teaspoon of gram flour and half teaspoon each of lime and cucumber juice. Apply daily 15 minutes before taking your bath till you are cured of your scars. Another effective method of removing scars is to apply for 10 minutes one-fourth teaspoon juices of lime, tomato and cucumber mixed together. Bleach the skin every week by taking one and a half teaspoon bleaching powder, one teaspoon hydrogen peroxide, four drops of liquid ammonia, a few drops of glycerine, and one teaspoon rose water. Mix the ingredients and leave on the face for 20 minutes. Besides, the importance of eating correct food cannot be overemphasised. Keep away from highly spiced and greasy foods because they stimulate secretion of oils. Also avoid eating sweet and starchy foods, nuts, etc. Fresh fruits and vegetables, cottage cheese, milk, lean meat, honey and plenty of water should go on top of your list.

It is very essential to keep your bowels clean because

constipation aggravates pimples. If necessary, take a mild laxative every other day. First thing in the morning, drink a glass of warm water to which juice of a lime has been added. This helps in clearing the blood-stream and, therefore, clears the skin of its blemishes and at the same time helps to work the bowels.

Chronic infection of teeth, tonsils, anaemia, dandruff, constipation, menstrual and glandular disturbances also play a major part in giving rise to pimples. Therefore, have yourself checked by your physician for your general health. Lastly, spend some time in the sun daily because sun's rays prove very beneficial in treating pimples. Go for walks in the evenings and develop a cheerful outlook. Brooding, depression and other emotional disturbances have a reaction on the skin. Also, sufficient sleep and exercise are good for general health and will help a great deal in combating acne.

Open Pores

To cure yourself of this condition, steam your face once a week with hot water to which juice of one lime and a teaspoon of rose water has been added. After about 10 minutes fill another basin with warm water. Add about 12 drops of tincture of benzoin to this. Bathe your face with this and then rub ice on the whole face. Pat dry, apply a little home-made cold cream. They are usually caused by excessive use of cream, Therefore, use liquid foundation and apply cucumber juice or lime juice blended with iced water to your face. When it dries completely, only then put on your makeup. The best remedy for enlarged pores is to daily rub on the skin half teaspoonful of lemon juice blended with one quarter teaspoonful each of milk and tomato juice.

Dark Lips

Heavy application of lipstick or the use of a cheap brand of lipstick turns the lips dark. Fresh air, vitamins and iron are required for maintaining red lips. Also keep them free from lipstick as much as possible and eat plenty of fruits and vegetables. Also, take carrot and orange juice. Every day before going to bed massage your lips with a few drops each of glycerine, lime juice and honey.

Freckles

These are exceedingly common pigmented spots of the skin which are frequently grouped or in rare cases scattered all over the surface of the body. They represent a reaction of the skin to the sun and will not appear if the skin is protected effectively from the sun. Sensitive skins are more prone to get freckles. Therefore, if you have a sensitive skin, never go out during the day without applying sun-screen lotion or cream to the face. If, however, you have already got freckles, every day an hour before you take your bath, take a teaspoon of finely-grated radish and mix with half teaspoon each of buttermilk and lime juice. This will remove superficial deposit of pigment, thus making many of the freckles disappear and make the others appear less prominent.

Prickly Heat

This is a very common condition during the hot days. The most effective remedy for treating prickly heat is to take a small piece of sandalwood and rub it to a paste on a stone with little rose water. Mix in a pinch of powdered alum and apply on the affected areas twice a day. To treat prickly heat in infants, dissolve a tablespoon of soda bicarbonate in half cup water. Mix in one teaspoon of rose water and apply on the affected portion a few times daily with cotton-wool.

During hot weather, small babies are troubled with boils on their heads. To remove them, scatter *neem* leaves on the baby's pillow. Once a week boil the leaves in a bucket of water for 15 minutes, cool the water, strain and give the baby his head-bath with this water.

Sunburns

They are caused when the skin is overexposed to the hot rays of the sun The symptoms vary with the intensity of the burns. The symptom may be just a slight flush or even blistering and loss of skin. Immediately after the burn, there may be a sensation of heat which is followed in a few days by itching and peeling of the skin. Sunburns seldom produce scars unless there is secondary infection of the damaged area. The application of vaseline or olive oil will stop the sensation of burning and dryness. In severe cases apply medication for burns to the affected areas.

Suntan

This is another skin ailment caused by the over-exposure of skin to the sun. The best remedy for removing suntan is to dip a piece of muslin in sour buttermilk and swathe your face in it for five minutes. Do this for 15 minutes and then wash off with water. Another remedy for sunburns is to take a tablespoon of buttermilk and mix in a teaspoon of tomato puree. Apply it on any portion of your body which has been affected by sunburns and wash off after half an hour with water.

Scars

To remove minor scars resulting from burns, take a small piece of dry coconut and hold it on fire with a pair of tongs until it turns black. Grind it and squeeze out its oil. Apply this oil a couple of times daily on the scars. it is very effective if applied on the skin immediately after the burn.

Scars resulting from these dreadful diseases often leave permanent disfigurement. But with a little care and attention they can be got rid of. However, you can ensure yourself of perfect results only if you take the treatments mentioned below immediately after you recover from this illness. You should keep in mind a few things if through some ill-luck you happen to fall a victim to it. Do not try to scratch any portion of your body during the illness or when you are recovering from it because due to constant scratching the scabs formed over the dried-up sores break giving rise to unsightly blemishes, which, if not treated, immediately can taint you for the rest of your life.

Abstain from salt and chillies completely during this period because it is mostly a salty and pungent diet which gives rise to an itchy sensation. After you have recovered completely that is, when all the scabs drop off, take a small lump of sugar candy (*khadi shakur*) and soak it in a small quantity of water overnight. Next morning, drain the water from it and keep it in a clean bowl. Now take the sugar candy and grind to a smooth paste. Add this paste to the water in the bowl. Apply it liberally over your entire face. Remove with water two hours after application. Besides, massage your face twice a weak nicely with home-made nourshing cream. After 10 minutes, remove all traces with cotton-wool and then take one tablespoon each of bleaching powder and hydrogen peroxide. Mix in five drops each of liquid ammonia, glycerine and rose water. Apply on the face and remove after 20 minutes with icy water. This treatment, if taken regularly, will slowly but surely give improvement.

Patches on the Skin

Patches are either dark or light in colour. The light ones can be cured by taking a little mustard oil and rubbing it vigorously on to the patch. Leave it on for a few hours before washing off with water. Do this twice a day. Also juices of both ribbed gourd (*toorai*) and basil (*tulsi*) are also effective in getting rid of these patches. Also, increase your intake of food rich in calcium. Supplement your diet with calcium tablets.

Dark patches can be eased away by rubbing on them a mixture of lime, tomato and cucumber juices. Take foods rich in vitamin B group. Supplement the daily diet with tablets of vitamin B.

Unwanted Hair

Hair covers the real beauty of a woman's skin making her feel self-conscious, but you can easily get rid of them. Here are a few methods by which you can get rid of unwanted hair. Adopt the one you find most suitable to you. Every one has some hair on the face; mostly it is a downy growth like the fuzz of a peach and this by no means is ugly. Still, if you feel you want to get rid of them, then the best thing is to bleach them which will make them almost unnoticeable. To one tablespoon of hydrogen add a few drops of liquid ammonia. Apply this mixture on your face with a piece of cotton-wool wrapped around an orange stick. Leave it on for about 10 minutes or until the hair turns golden. Then, rinse thoroughly with cold water. You can bleach the hair three or four times a month depending upon when your hair turns black.

Before starting on bleaching, you should keep a few points in mind. When bleaching your face, keep the mixture well away from your eyes. Avoid any small cuts or grazes because it will make them sting. Never bleach a pimply face. If your skin is on the sensitive side apply a little of it on the inside of your wrist (before using the bleach) to see whether it agrees with your skin. If it does not agree, never go in for bleaching.

If you have a dry skin, then, before bleaching, apply a thin layer of cold cream on your face. Bleaching can be used with advantage on the hair on the stomach and around the nipples. If the hair on these regions happen to be long, cut them short with scissors before bleaching them. But on no account use any other treatment on these regions.

Another remedy for hair on the face is to use home-made hair-removing cream. To prepare it take one kilo. *masoor dal* (red gram pulse), $\frac{1}{4}$ kilo. dried orange peels, two well-beaten eggs and coconut water. Soak *dal* in water for one day. Dry in the sun, mix in the eggs and dry again nicely in the sun. Grind both the *dal* and peels to a paste and store in airtight tin. Every day take two tablespoons of this mixture and put in enough water to form a thin paste. Apply on the face. When it feels a little dry, start rubbing your face vigorously with your hands till all the paste falls off. Remove the paste which still clings on with water. If this treatment is taken regularly, it will not only remove unwanted hair and all the blemishes but will at the same time make the skin petal soft and silky smooth.

But on no case use a razor or hair-removing creams or wax on your face, because these give rise to coarse open pores, black patches and a coarse hair growth. They make the hair grow twice as fast and twice as thick as it would be otherwise.

The only effective treatment for a thick growth of hair on arms and legs is to use home-made wax on them. This is a treatment which is simple and highly effective, because it takes away the hair from its roots. Subsequent re-growth is thus weakened and discouraged and the growing-in period becomes longer every time. Apply a thick layer of wax with a blunt knife in the direction of the hair. Place a strip of cotton cloth over it. Then press down on all the sides for a firm grip. Holding the lower end of the cloth pull off with a firm sweeping movement in the direction opposite to your growth. When the cloth is full of hair, discard it and use a fresh clean one. Use this method after every 25 or 30 days.

Daily rubbing the affected area with a pumice stone after waxing the hair away first keeps the hair from protruding beyond the surface of the skin. In many cases, the continuous use of this method is known to have considerably lessened the growth. The best way to use this stone is to lather up the skin with soap and water and use it in a circular motion on the area to be 'defuzzed'.

Hair disappears by friction. Wash off with water and finally apply a little olive oil over the area.

Skin Allergy

Skin allergy means that one is more sensitive to some particular substance than others. Allergies are caused by anything from food, cosmetics, clothing, fibres, pollen, plants and even animals. Cosmetic allergy is manifested by skin eruptions, swelling of tissues, itching and many others symptoms. If you find that you are breaking out into any of the above-mentioned symptoms and discover that you have used a new lipstick, powder or cream then you should eliminate the encounter with the offending agent immediately. The symptoms of food allergy are belching, nauses, vomiting, abdominal pain, constipation or diarrhea, sores around the mouth and the swelling of the lips, tongue or throat. Trial diets in which suspected foods are eliminated one by one are particularly helpful in furnishing clues to the allergy. Your doctor can give you a prescription to alleviate the reaction but once you know what the encounter with the culprit does to you, avoid it as plague and remember that you can suddenly develop an allergy to a substance which you have been using or taking for a long time; therefore, suspect everything unless you find out the real 'culprit'.

8

Beauty Aids From Natural Ingredients

THERE ARE cosmetics bearing well-known trade marks used by most women today. But there also exist certain beauty aids made from natural ingredients, which were in vogue in this country a few decades ago and are still used by intelligent women.

The Indispensable Lime

This well known citrus fruit so commonly used hardly needs any introduction. This cheap golden-coloured fruit has excellent properties which can help you to become lovely by enhancing your good looks and improving your figure.

1. *For very oily skin*, sqeeze lemon juice in a bowl of iced water. Splash this over the face, massage for five minutes and then wash off with water.

2. *To relieve tired eyes*, take four tablespoons each of lime juice and iced water. Saturate cotton pads in this water and place over your closed eyelides for 10 minutes.

3. *To improve a dull and greasy complexion*, mix half teaspoon of lime juice with one teaspoon of cucumber juice and a few drops of rose water. Apply on the face and neck and leave on for 15 minutes then remove with water.

4. *To shrink open pores*, apply lime juice on the pores

on the skin and rinse after 15 minutes.

5. *For falling hair*, squeeze out the juice of a lime and mix with four tablespoons of thick coconut milk. Rub well into the scalp and let it remain for one hour. Repeat it once a week till you effect a cure.

6. *To improve a dry and rough skin*, take an egg yolk and mix in a few drops of lime and olive oil. Spread on the face and leave it till the skin feels dry. Wash off with ordinary water and splash on cold water.

7. *To lighten your complexion*, take one teaspoon each of lime, cucumber and carrot juice. Apply on the face and leave on for 15 minutes before washing off with water.

8. *To put a sparkle in your teeth*, clean them once a week with lime juice to which little salt has been added.

9. *To remove sun-tan*, apply lime juice mixed with little rose water on the face before going to bed in the night. Next morning, wash off with water.

10. *To remove lice from the head*, take two tablespoons of lemon juice and mix in equal quantity of ginger juice. Rub it gently in the scalp in the night and tie a muslin round your head. Next morning take your head-bath.

11. *To remove freckles*, blanch and grind two almonds and mix with white of an egg to which half teaspoon of lime juice has been added. Spread on the face and leave on till the skin feels dry. Then, wash off first with warm water and then with cold water.

12. *To care a blemished skin*, mix two tablespoons of pureed prunes with one teaspoon of lime juice and eat half an hour before going to bed. On this drink a glass of warm water.

13. *Plenty of lime juice* should be taken each day because the ascorbic acid content of lime helps in the

quicker healing of wounds, helps maintain your teeth, hair, nails and complexion in good condition and guards you against catching colds.

Oils for Beauty

For enhancing your good looks there is nothing like the ordinary oil. Here are a few inexpensive beauty tips which will help you maintain a flawless complexion.

1. In very cold weather prevent the *chapping of your skin* by taking a teaspoon of castor oil and mixing with it half a teaspoon of rose water. Apply on the face and neck in the night and remove it first thing in the morning.

2. To counteract *sun-tan*, mix olive oil with equal quantity of vinegar and apply the mixture an hour before you take your bath.

3. For counteracting a *dry skin*, soak a muslin cloth in warm olive oil and cover your face with it after making holes for the eyes and nose. Let it remain for half an hour and then wipe the face with a soft cloth. Let the face remain as it is the whole night. Next morning, wash it with warm water and splash on cold water.

4. An *anti-wrinkle cream* is made by mixing a teaspoon of olive oil with an egg. Smoothen the face and neck with it and let it remain till the skin gets dry. Then, remove it with a piece of cotton-wool dipped in hot water to which a teaspoon of soda bicarbonate has been added.

5. The best *beauty mask* can be made by mixing a tablespoon of gram flour with one-fourth teaspoon of orange peel powder, one tablespoon of beaten curd and one teaspoon of olive oil. Mix well and apply the paste to your

face and neck. Let it remain till the skin starts feeling a little dry and then rub your face with your hands till it glows. Wash your face first with warm and then cold water. This removes all the emarrassing blemishes from the skin and makes it soft and smooth.

6. To improve *a blemished and discloured face*, first steam it for 10 minutes. Clean your face with a cleanser, wipe dry with a soft napkin and then apply a teaspoon of olive oil mixed with half a teaspoon of lime juice. Let it remain for 20 minutes, wipe with cotton-wool and rub ice cube gently for five minutes over the face.

7. To improve a *dark and dull complexion*, mix a teaspoon of gram flour to which a pinch of turmeric powder, a few drops of lime juice and half a teaspoon each of olive oil and milk has been added. Leave on for half an hour and then wash off with water.

8. Improve *weak nails* by applying baby oil mixed with white iodine on the nails and base of culticles every day.

9. For *lined and chapped lips* the best remedy is to massage them daily at bedtime with baby oil.

10. Brush pure castor oil on the roots of your *lashes* at bedtime to make them grow long and thick.

11. Massage *grey and wrinkled elbows* every day at bedtime with baby oil to make them soft and smooth.

12. Massage your *face and neck* every night at bedtime with baby oil to make it soft, smooth, glowing.

13. If the *skin around your heels* has become hard and cracked, scrub your heels with a stiff brush using soap generously. Then rub them nicely with pumice stone. Wash with water, wipe dry and then massage nicely with castor oil.

14. To improve *rough and dry complexion* take a teaspoon of almond oil and mix with half a teaspoon each of cream milk and lime juice. Apply every night before going to bed both on the face and on the neck.

15. An excellent cleaner for a *dry skin* is made by mixing yolk of an egg with half a teaspoon of olive oil and a few drops of lime juice. Apply on face and neck. Leave on for 15 minutes and wash first with warm and then with cold water.

16. To cure yourself of *dry, itchy skin* take cod-liver oil at the rate of one teaspoon a day for one whole month.

17. To treat *rough, dry skin* around knees, elbows and heels massage these areas regularly with a paste made of salt and mustard oil.

18. In the *cold weather*, take oil bath to prevent your body from becoming rough and dry. Put two tablespoons of olive oil in your bath water along with a few drops of your favourite Cologne. Your skin will turn soft and glowing after you have had your bath.

Beauty from Leaves

Many effective beauty aids are made from ordinary leaves. Here are some of them which will help you to maintain a flawless complexion.

Celery leaves—Clean, slice and boil a couple of handfuls of celery leaves in a small bucket of water. Remove from fire, cool and strain the water. Mix in a tablespoon of vinegar. Rinse your hair after shampooing with this water and see how your hair grows long and lustrous.

Leaves of ribbed gourd—Clean, slice and grind the leaves of this vegetable to a paste and apply over dark patches (on your body) left-over from some skin disease a few times daily. Within a week the patches will vanish, leaving no trace behind.

Bilva leaves—These are green leaves used in the worship of Lord Shiva. If you are suffering from offensive body odour, grind a handful of these leaves to a paste and apply this paste all over your body half an hour before going in for your bath. Do this twice a week till you effect a cure.

Bay leaves—If you want to make your teeth sparkle, rub them twice a week with a dry bay leaf and see how women envy your bright smile.

Lettuce leaves—Grind a lettuce leaf with a small rose to a paste and mix in a few drops of lime juice. Apply this paste over your face and leave it on for 15 minutes. Remove with water. This is excellent for counteracting a greasy skin.

Mint leaves—Wash and grind a few mint leaves to a smooth paste. Apply over your face every night before you go to sleep. This helps you to get rid of pimples and other embarrassing blemishes of the skin.

Mehandi or henna leaves—These leaves are being used for centuries in India by women to dye their hair and to decorate their palms and feet. You can have best results if you soak fresh leaves for a whole night in water. The following morning drain out the water and grind them to a paste with a little *kattha* (used in *pan*), some lime juice, sugar and turmeric powder. This way, the colour of the *mehandi* will come out bright red. They are also used for darkening the hair and encouraging their growth. Soak a few *amlas* (Indian gooseberrys) in a little milk for a couple of hours and then grind them to a smooth paste along with a handful of *mehandi* leaves.

Mix well and rub into the roots of hair an hour before you go in for your headbath.

Neem leaves—These leaves are very useful for removing scars from the body caused by chickenpox and smallpox. They also help in the case of small boils, itching and prickly heat. Boil a couple of handfuls of these leaves in a bucket of water till the water is reduced to three-fourths its original quantity. Remove the water from fire, cool and strain and let the patient use it in his bath and within a week you will find a definite improvement in his condition.

Tea leaves—Left-over tea leaves are very good for preventing the hair from falling and they also make the hair glossy and soft. Therefore, next time do not throw away used tea leaves, use them for washing your hair. Put the leaves in a bucket of water and boil for 15 minutes. Remove from fire, cool and strain and use this for washing your hair instead of ordinary water. If lime juice is added to this water and it is used as a last rinse, it gives a lustrous sheen to the hair.

These leaves are also excellent for reviving tired eyes. Mix some crushed ice in used tea leaves. Tie them up in two small pieces of cloth and put them on each eyelid for 10 minutes. They will not only remove tiredness from the eyes but will also make them brighter. They are also very good for treating sunburns. Dissolve four teaspoons tea leaves in boiling water. Strain and mix with clear, greasy surgical jelly and place in airtight jar.

Tulsi leaves—The leaves of Indian basil *tulsi* are very beneficial to the human body. Make a habit of taking a teaspoon of these leaves mixed with honey once a day to put a glow in your cheeks and to keep all the diseases away. This juice is also very effective for getting rid of lice. Apply it liberally to the head in the night and cover it with a towel. Next morning, wash your head in the usual way. Do this for a few weeks to effect a cure. If your baby has lice, scatter them on his pillow for a couple of days.

These leaves also help in cases of almost all the skin diseases and removal of patches from the skin. Grind them to a paste and apply to the affected portions of the skin a few times daily for a few days and you will be completely relieved of your ailment. These leaves help even when all the other medicines have failed. It is rightly said—'A *tulsi* leaf a day keeps all diseases and skin ailments away'.

Beauty from Milk

To make your skin *soft and smooth* dip a piece of cotton-wool in milk and pat all over your face. Leave on for half an hour and wash off with water.

Mix two tablespoons of milk in one teaspoon of salt and apply on the face at bedtime. This makes the skin *petal-soft and silken-smooth.*

To *lighten your complexion* grind a couple of almonds in milk and apply on the face at bedtime.

To *brighten a dull complexion* mix two tablespoons of milk powder with enough hydrogen peroxide to a thick paste. Mix in a few drops of liquid ammonia. Leave on for 15 minutes.

To *improve a dark and dull complexion* soak *chana dal* in milk overnight. Next morning, grind to a paste and mix in a pinch of turmeric powder and a few drops of lime juice and leave on for half an hour.

To *lighten and brighten your complexion* take a tablespoon of milk and mix in one teaspoon each of carrot, orange juice and melted honey. Leave it on for 15 minutes.

An excellent *mask for a dry and blemished skin* is made by taking a tablespoon of gram flour and mixing in a big pinch of turmeric powder, one-fourth teaspoon of orange peel powder, a teaspoon of beaten curd and a teaspoon of milk. Apply on the face and neck. When the skin starts feeling taut, rub it with your hands until it glows. Then, wash with tap water.

To make the skin *soft and smooth* grind one-fourth teaspoon of *chironji* to a paste and mix with one-fourth teaspoon each of milk and curd. Leave on for 20 minutes.

Another *mask for making the skin soft and smooth* is prepared by taking one-fourth teaspoon each of watermelon, cucumberand gourd seeds and grinding them to a paste in milk. Mix in half teaspoon of cream or top of milk and a few drops of rose water. Leave on for 20 minutes.

To *lighten and brighten the skin and improve blood circulation* fry a teaspoon of *masoor dal* in a teaspoon of olive oil to a red colour, grind to a paste in milk. Apply on face and leave on till the skin feels taut. Then, rub the skin till it glows and wash off.

For making the *skin fair*, grind as small piece of sandlewood in milk to a paste. Mix in one-fourth teaspoon of turmeric powder and leave on for 20 minutes.

To *remove itching and other blemishes* from the skin grind one teaspoon of yellow mustard to a paste and mix with a tablespoon of cream of milk and leave on for 20 minutes.

To *improve a dry and rough skin* take two tablespoon cream of milk and add a teaspoon of almond oil and a few drops of essence of rose. Leave on for half an hour before removing with water. Besides using milk externally, drink a glass every day in order to keep your teeth, hair, nails and eyes in good condition and to put a glow into your face.

Beauty from Vegetables and Fruits

Highly effective facepacks and lotions can be prepared from fruits and vegetables which will give your skin a soft, lovely radiance.

Astringent lotion—Blanch a small peach, remove its stone and grind and squeeze out its juice. Add to it one-fourth teaspoon each of lime and tomato juice. Mix well and spread on your face and neck and leave on for 15 minutes.

Cucumber tonic—Grate and squeeze out juice from a small cucumber and mix in one-fourth teaspoon each of lime juice and rose water. Apply on face and leave on for 15 minutes. This tonic improves a dull and greasy complexion.

Cleansing lotion—To one-fourth teaspoon of lime juice stir in one teaspoon each of milk and cucumber juice. Apply on the face and neck and wash off after 14 minutes. This lotion cleanses and purifies the pores of the skin.

Cabbage mask—Grind a couple of cabbage leaves and extract juice. Dissolve one-fourth teaspoon of yeast in it and stir in one teaspoon of honey. Mix well and apply thickly over face and neck. Remove with cotton-wool soaked in water 15 minutes after application. This mask will counteract any tendency towards wrinkles and dryness and give your skin a flower-like bloom.

Orange tonic—Blanch and grind a couple of almonds to a paste and mix in two tablespoons of milk and one tablespoon each of carrot and orange juice. Apply thickly on face and neck and leave on for half an hour. Removes scars and blemishes from the face and makes it soft and smooth.

Tomato lotion—To one tablespoon of tomato juice add a couple of drops of lime juice. Apply on face and remove after 15 minutes. It is very effective for shrinking enlarged pores.

Watermelon lotion—Grate and squeeze out juice from a small piece of watermelon. Apply on face and neck and leave on for 15 minutes. This lotion freshens up the skin.

Whitening lotion—To one tablespoon of cucumber juice stir in a few drops of lime juice and a dash of turmeric powder. Apply on face and neck and wash off after half an hour. Makes an excellent whitener for all types of skins.

Potato tonic—Grind and squeeze juice of potatoes. Apply on face and neck and leave on whole night. Next morning, wash with water to which a little witch-hazel has been added. This tonic whitens and brightens the skin.

Carrot lotion—To one-fourth teaspoon of carrot juice add one teaspoon of melted honey. Remove with cotton-wool soaked in water to which a little soda bicarbonate has been added after 15 minutes. It removes roughness from the skin and makes it smooth as silk.

Tomato tonic—To two teaspoons of tomato juice add four tablespoons of buttermilk. Remove after half an hour. It is excellent for removing sunburns.

Cucumber lotion—One tablespoon each of cucumber juice and milk and a few drops of rose water should be mixed together and applied on the face and neck and removed after 15 minutes. Makes excellent whitener for delicate skins.

Grape lotion—One tablespoon grape juice should be applied on the face and neck and left on for 15 minutes. Makes the skin soft and smooth, bright and fair.

Papaya cream—Apply one tablespoon finely ground raw papaya to the face and leave on for 15 minutes. Removes pimples and other embarrassing blemishes.

Apple tonic—Mix one tablespoon of apple juice with one-fourth teaspoon of lime juice. Leave on for 20 minutes. Makes excellent tonic for combating greasiness.

Coconut lotion—Water of coconut, if rubbed on the skin and left on for 15 minutes, lightens and brightens the skin.

9

How to Stay Slim

ARE YOU one of those perennial dieters who loses 10, 15 or even 20 pounds but never seems able to keep them lost ? This is because many people soon get tired of continuous semi-starvation and therefore once again they start eating a full diet and than they are right back where they started. Whatever method you try in becoming slim you will not achieve success unless you keep down the intake of food. If you think it is worth the effort to remain slim for looks, for health reasons and to please your better half, start dieting from today and establishing new food habits. You think it is hard ? Not at all. Here are a few simple rules which will tell you how to diet the easy way. If you follow them faithfully, they will surely give birth to a 'newer you' in no time.

1. Face up to the fact that the first few weeks of dieting are going to be tough on your stomach because going on a diet means that you have got to eat much less than you usually eat, which means all the time you are going to feel gnawing in your tummy. Whenever you feel the craving for food, that is the time when the fat is literally and actually disappearing. So, teach yourself to regard these pangs of hunger as the birth pangs of a 'new you'. In the beginning your body will protest, but soon it will stop when it realises that you mean business.

In order to train your body to eat less, you must keep busy constantly. If you sit at home doing nothing, naturally you will find that the only diversion you have from your boredom is to eat. Therefore, if you have no work then develop a hobby. Spend the money you usually use to gorge yourself with food on your favourite hobby. Some people, who are reducing, find that reading or going to the movies are acceptable substitutes. Others find substitutes in writing, embroidery, painting, stitching, etc. Once you keep yourself busily occupied your mind will have no time to dwell upon food.

2. Substitute low calorie foods for higher ones. Lean meat, fish, chicken, eggs, skim milk, cottage cheese, fruits and vegetables are for you. Cut down on all the heavy desserts except desserts made with gelatin, honey and fresh fruits. But of course you will not like to eat the non-fattening foods for the first fortnight or so, but slowly and steadily you will develop a taste for them. Once you get used to your new diet, you will reduce by leaps and bounds.

3. For the first few weeks try not to eat with the others at the table because naturally the tantalising rich smell of their food will tempt you. Therefore, in the beginning eat by yourself or at a different time from the rest of the household.

4. Take some sort of exercise daily. Go for long brisk walks in the mornings and in the evenings. Play tennis, play with your children, swim and cycle. Do anything but do not keep sitting at one place for any length of time. Keep on the move. This is good for your health and your figure.

5. Keep a weekly diary of your weight and essential measurements. Weigh yourself on a reliable scale. Never weigh yourself more than once because the weight varies from hour to hour and the varying message of the scale might weigh on your mind and make you depressed.

For example, in the morning your weight is normally less than the evening, because your stomach is empty and the fluid which has left the body may weigh a half pound or thereabouts and so you will weigh less for a short time; but in the evenings you will weigh one or two pounds more. In the same way, the weight varies from day to day because of the varying amount of water the body retains in the different cells and in the bladder. Therefore, a little increase in weight should not alarm you. Weigh yourself preferably in the morning, in the same clothes, always on the same scale and on the same day the next week.

Once you have lost your weight do not again start gorging yourself on rich and heavy foods which will prove suicidal to dieting. You can eat an occasional rich food a few times a month once you have been able to maintain your weight without losing everything, but remember a dieter must learn to live with temptations all her life.

Seven-day Menu for Reducing

FIRST DAY

Breakfast

First thing in the morning, take one cup warm water to which strained juice of a lime and one teaspoon of honey has been added. This helps in clearing the bloodstream and therefore clears the skin of its blemishes and at the same time helps to work the bowels. Therefore, make it a 'religious' duty to drink this daily. Later on for breakfast take one cup of skimmed milk, one boiled egg, one thin slice of brown bread spread upon with one tsp. butter, one apple, one fish liver oil capsule for vitamin A and D, 100 miligram vitamin C tablet and six brewers yeast tablets containing the entire B family. Take these vitamins also daily in the morning without fail.

Lunch

Mutton stew; Spinach delight; Raita; One chapati; One orange.

To prepare mutton stew, take 250 gram lean mutton, 100 gram mixed vegetables (tomatoes, carrots, peas and french beans) one-quarter coconut, a few each of mint and curry leaves, one small onion, salt and spices to taste. Grind coconut and extract juice. Set this thick juice aside. Pour one cup hot water on the squeezed out coconut scrapings and set aside for five minutes. Then squeeze out the milk. This is known as thin milk. Put mutton, salt and spices in this thin milk and cook till almost tender, put in the vegetables and mint leaves and continue cooking till both the mutton and vegetables are done. Fry onion and curry leaves in half a teaspoon of oil to a light brown colour, pour over the stew and serve at once.

To prepare spinach delight, take half a cup of chopped spinach, quarter cup skimmed milk, half a tablespoon powdered cumin seeds, salt to taste, half a tablespoon sliced ginger, one minced green chilli.

Put the spinach to cook with chilli and salt and ginger. Let it get cooked thoroughly and allow the water to dry. Mash to a paste, put in the milk, re-heat and sprinkle cumin seeds on top.

For raita, take half cup curd made out of milk with cream removed, two tablespoons grated and steamed marrow of pumpkin, a few corriander leaves, quarter tablespoon grated ginger, salt and spices to taste.

Beat the curd well and mix in the marrow with the rest of the things.

Tea time

One glass of tomato juice.

Dinner

Two cups soup, two melba toasts and fruit salad.

For soup, take $\frac{1}{4}$ chicken without skin, one egg, one slice of pomfret, 100 gram. mixed vegetables (french beans, peas, cabbage, carrots), salt and soya sauce to taste. Beat the egg lightly. Steam-cook the vegetables and fish. Flake the fish and chop the vegetables. Boil chicken in two glasses of water. When tender, strain out the soup and remove the chicken from the bones. Mix chicken soup and soya sauce into the egg and stir well. Put in the vegetables and fish and serve at once.

For melba toast, lay 2 brown breads on a shallow baking tray, place tray in a very slow oven and bake until perfectly dry and crisp. Spread each toast with half teaspoon butter.

For fruit salad, take one cup orange juice, $\frac{1}{2}$ cup diced mixed fruits of choice, one teaspoon gelatin and honey to suit the taste. Dissolve gelatin in one tablespoon warm water. Also dissolve honey in orange juice by placing both on slow fire Mix in gelatin. Remove from fire, cool, put in the fruits and chill.

Bed time

One cup of skimmed milk.

SECOND DAY

Breakfast

Drink the warm water, lime juice and honey mixture.

Later on take one scrambled egg, one slice of brown bread spread with half teaspoon butter, one orange. Also, take all the tablets mentioned above and one cup skimmed milk. Scramble the egg in half teaspoon butter only.

Lunch

Fish curry, chapati, one glass buttermilk, salad and 100 gram grapes. For fish curry, take two slices of pomfret, a large floweret cauliflower, 50 gram mixed vegetables (peas, french beans and carrots), half tablespoon grated ginger, one crushed garlic flake, one tablespoon curd, one small tomato, one small minced onion, $\frac{1}{4}$ tablespoon turmeric powder, $\frac{1}{4}$ tablespoon *garam masala*, salt to taste, a few corriander leaves and chilli powder to taste.

Apply salt and turmeric on fish and set aside for 15 minutes. Heat one tablespoon oil and fry ginger, garlic and onion, add tomato and curd and cook till dry, put in the vegetables and fry for five minutes. Pour one and a half cup hot water, add fish and cook till both vegetables and fish are done. Sprinkle corriander leaves and *garam masala* on top.

Salad : Mix together finely sliced raw carrot, beetroot, cucumber, tomato and onion and sprinkle overl lime juice, salt and pepper.

Tea time

Take one cup each of cucumber and carrot juice. Mix together and season with salt.

Dinner

Mutton cake, two melba toasts and orange sponge.

For mutton cake, take one cup minced mutton, one slice bread, one small tomato, half tablespoon grated ginger, one minced green chilli, a few corriander leaves, salt and spices to taste.

Soak bread in milk and squeeze dry, then mix into the mince along with the rest of the above ingredients. Put in a greased mould. Put the mould in a tray of hot water and bake in an oven till set. Serve with one poached egg and grilled tomato.

To poach the egg break it in a small greased bowl and steam over hot water till it turns firm.

Melba toasts should be made as shown above.

For orange sponge, take $\frac{3}{4}$ cup orange juice, one tablespoon gelatin, one egg white, stiffly beaten, two tablespoons honey.

Dissolve gelatin in one tablespoon hot water, add the juice and honey, warm the mixture till the honey dissolves then chill till partially set, beat in the egg white and chill till firm. Decorate with orange slices.

Bed time

One cup skimmed milk

THIRD DAY

Breakfast

Take warm water, lime juice and honey mixture. Besides take one poached egg, one slice brown bread spread with one teaspoon butter, one cup skimmed milk, one apple. Also take all the vitamins as shown in the breakfast of the first day.

Lunch

Cream cheese *bhaji*, one *roti*, baked potatoes, salad, one glass buttermilk.

Prepare cream cheese *bhaji* thus. Take ¼ litre milk, ¼ cup curd, one tablespoon lime juice. Besides, take one cup minced spinach, one small onion (minced), one green chilli, minced, one medium tomato (sliced), ¼ teaspoon turmaric powder, salt, chilli and spices to taste. Boil the milk and mix in beaten curd and lime juice. When the milk curds, strain through a cloth, tie it closely and hang it up to drip in a bowl until no more water flows. Then, place the cheese between two flat plates and place a heavy weight on the uppermost plate for half an hour. Remove the weight, plates and cloth and cut the cheese into small pieces. Now heat one tablespoon oil and fry the onion, ginger and chilli until soft. Add spinach, tomato, remaining spices and water that had dripped out of the cheese. Cook till the spinach is dry. Mash to a paste, put in one cup hot water and cheese and cook for five minutes.

Baked potatoes : Take a large potato cut in half and scoop out middle portion until only about half inch is left lining the skin. Rub with half tablespoon oil blended with salt and bake in very hot oven till brown and crisp.

Salad : Fix a plate with tender carrot sticks, bits of raw cauliflower, red and white radishes, tomatoes and cucumber and sprinkle on the top lime juice, salt and pepper.

Tea time

One glass carrot juice.

Dinner

Roast chickcn, two slices brown bread, fruit cup.

Roast chicken : Take one half kilo chicken and use it for two days. Besides, take 250 gram of mixed vegetables (carrots, french beans, cabbage and peas), one medium tomato (minced), one tablespoon grated ginger, one medium onion (minced), two green chillis (minced), ¼ teaspoon each of *garam masala* and turmeric powder, handful of corriander leaves, salt and chilli powder to taste.

Heat one teaspoon oil and fry the onion and ginger till soft. Add tomato along with the rest of the spices and cook till dry, add vegetables and fry for two minutes. Put in a quarter cup hot water and cook till the vegetables are almost tender and dry. Clean the chicken nicely and rub insides with salt and pepper, put in the stuffing, tie up, rub the outside with one teaspoon butter blended with salt and pepper and bake in a hot oven for one hour or till done.

Fruit cup : One cup curd made of skimmed milk, ½ cup sliced fruit of choice. Honey, chill curd, put alternate layers of fruits and curd in a glass with a layer of honey in between. Decorate the top with a slice of fruit.

Bed time

One cup skimmed milk.

FOURTH DAY

Breakfast

First thing in the morning, drink a cup of warm water to which lime juice, honey have been added. Later on take two boiled eggs, one sliced brown bread spread with a teaspoon of butter, one cup skimmed milk and all the vitamins as shown in the first day.

Lunch

Drumstick Maharajah, carrot salad, one *roti*, boiled fish, one orange.

Drumstick Maharajah : Two drumsticks, scraped and diced into pieces, ½ teaspoon grated ginger, ¼ teaspoon cumin seeds, a big pinch each of trumeric powder and *garam masala*, one medium tomato (sliced), one teaspoon corriander powder, a handful of corriander leaves, five tablespoons skimmed milk, one tablespoon tomato ketchup, salt and chilli powder to taste.

Heat one teaspoon oil and toss in cumin seeds and ginger. When the seeds stop popping, put in the tomato and all the spices and cook till soft. Mix in the drumsticks, milk and ketchup and corriander leaves and cook over a slow fire till soft and almost dry.

Carrot salad : One carrot (grated), two tablespoons *moong dal*, ¼ coconut (grated), a few corriander leaves, one chilli (minced), one tablespoon juice of lime, a big pinch mustard seeds. Soak whole *moong* in water for 12 hours, drain the water and tie in a wet cloth and set aside for 24 hours, at the end of which it developes sprouts. Heat one teaspoon oil and toss in mustard seeds. When they stop, add the *dal* and cook for two minutes, mix in the rest of the things with the exception of lime juice and remove from fire. Mix in the lime juice.

Boiled fish : Two slices pomfet, one small carrot (halved), pinch of nutmeg, one small onion (halved), a few peppercorns, salt and lime juice to taste. Put fish in one cup water along with spices, salt, carrot and onion and boil in water till soft and discard carrot and onion and peppercorns. Squeeze juice and, if you like, put tomato ketchup over the fish.

Dinner

Left-over roast chicken as made on the previous day, two slices of brown bread, mixed fruit delight.

Mixed fruit delight : Take 200 gram of mixed dry fruits like prunes, apricots and raisins. Cover them with warm water and two tablespoons honey and let them stand thus for 24 hours.

Bed time

One cup skimmed milk.

FIFTH DAY

Breakfast

Take lime juice, warm water and honey mixture. Later on take two boiled eggs, one melba toast spread with one teaspoon butter, one cup skimmed milk. Also take all the vitamins as shown on the first day.

Lunch

Stuffed capsicum, grilled liver. one orange, one *roti*, one glass buttermilk.

Stuffed capsicum : Two medium capsicums, 150 gram minced lean mutton, one small onion (minced), one green chilli (minced), handful of corriander leaves, $\frac{1}{2}$ teaspoon grated ginger, salt and spices to taste, one tablespoon tomato ketchup. Cut out half inch from the top of capsicums. Mix all the mutton mixture together with the exception of ketchup. Scoop out the seeds from the capsicums. Fill with meat mixture and place in baking dish. Mix ketchup with $\frac{1}{4}$ cup warm water and pour over the capsicums. Bake in a moderate oven till done basting frequently.

Grilled liver : Take $\frac{1}{2}$ liver, cut into square pieces, salt and spices to taste. Mix salt and spices in one teaspoon oil and rub over liver. Place on oiled grill and grill till tender. Sprinkle lime juice on top.

Tea time

One glass tomato juice.

Dinner

Coconut custard, clear soup, two slices brown bread, baked fish.

Coconut custard : $\frac{1}{2}$ cup thick coconut milk, two tablespoons grated jaggery, one egg (beaten), a big pinch nutmeg. Dissolve jaggery in milk. Mix in the rest of the ingredients, put in a greased mould and steam till set.

Soup : Boil two glasses of water. Mix vegetables of choice. Remove from fire, strain out the soup, re-heat, put in salt, pepper and lime juice and if you like a crumbled egg yolk left-over from breakfast.

Baked fish : Two slices pomfret, two tablespoons milk, one teaspoon butter, crumbs, salt and spices to taste. Rub salt and spices on fish. Dip in milk, roll lightly in crumbs and put in a greased baking dish. Dot with butter and bake in a very hot oven on both the sides till brown and crisp.

Bed time

One cup skimmed milk.

SIXTH DAY

Take warm water, lime juice and honey mixture Later on take one poached egg, one brown bread slice spread with one teaspoon butter, one apple, one cup skimmed milk. Also take all the vitamins as shown on the first day.

Lunch

One *roti*, cream cheese with fenugreek leaves, vegetable stew, one glass buttermilk.

Cream cheese with fenugreek leaves : Make cream cheese as shown in the lunch recipes of third day. Besides take one cup fenugreek leaves, one chilli (minced), one medium tomato (sliced), a few corriander leaves, $\frac{1}{4}$ teaspoon turmeric powder, one teaspoon corriander powder, a big pinch *garam masala*, salt and chilli powder to taste. Heat one teaspoon oil and put all the spices, leaves and tomato, chilli and corriander leaves. When the leaves are tender and quite dry, mix in the cheese and remove from fire.

Vegetable stew : 250 gram. mixed vegetables (french beans, carrots, cauliflower, peas and lady fingers), one big tomato, one teaspoon grated ginger, two green chillis (minceed), $\frac{1}{2}$ teaspoon cumin seeds, $\frac{1}{2}$ teaspoon turmeric powder, handful of corriander leaves, salt and other spices to taste. Heat one teaspoon *ghee* or oil and add cumin seeds and ginger. When the seeds stop popping, add all the spices, chillis, corriander leaves and tomato. When the tomato turns soft and dry, put in all the vegetables. Mix well and then put in one and a half cup water. When the vegetables are cooked, remove from fire. Do not put lady fingers with other vegetables. Put them in when the other vegetables are half cooked.

Tea time

One cup pineapple juice mixed with one cup of beet-root juice.

Dinner

Irish stew, apple delight, two slices of brown bread.

Irish stew : 250 gram. lean mutton, 150 gram. mixed vegetables (carrots, tomatoes, baby onions, frenchbeans, cabbage, peas), two teablespoons sliced celeray, salt and pepper to taste. Put a layer of mutton and vegetables in a heavy saucepan till all the ingredients have been used up. Cover with warm water and cook till both the mutton and vegetables are done.

Apple delight : One teaspoon butter, one finely shredded apple, honey to taste, two finely sliced almonds. Heat butter till it melts. Put in apple and heat thoroughly. Sprinkle with honey and almonds.

Bed time

One cup skimmed milk.

SEVENTH DAY

Breakfast

Take lime juice, warm water and honey mixture. Later on take one poached egg, one slice of toast spread with one teaspoon butter, one cup skimmed milk, 100 gram. grapes, and one orange. Besides, take all the vitamins as listed in the first day's breakfast.

Lunch

Cream cheese in tomato, *raita*, one *roti*, baked potatoes as shown under THIRD DAY.

Cream cheese in tomato : Make the cheese in the same way as in the lunch recipes of the THIRD DAY. Besides, take one big tomato (sliced), one chilli (minced), a few corriander leaves, $\frac{1}{4}$ teaspoon turmeric powder, one teaspoon grated ginger, a big pinch cumin seeds, salt and spices to taste. Heat one teaspoon oil and put in the cumin seeds and ginger. When the seeds stop popping, add tomato along with all the ingredients with the exception of cheese. Cook till dry, add one cup warm water, put in the cheese and cook for five minutes more.

Raita : One cup curd made of skimmed milk, 50 gram mixed steamed vegetables (french beans, carrots, peas) one cucumber (grated), one chilli (minced), $\frac{1}{4}$ inch ginger (grated), a few mint leaves, $\frac{1}{2}$ teaspoon roasted and ground cumin seeds, salt and pepper to taste. Mix everything together.

Tea time

One glass tomato juice.

Dinner

Two slices bread, chutney fish, soup as prepared in SIXTH DAY's dinner recipes, salad, fruit salad as prepared for FIRST DAY.

Chutney fish : Two slices pomfret, $\frac{1}{4}$ cup corriander leaves, two green chillis, $\frac{1}{4}$ teaspoon cumin seeds, one flake garlic, $\frac{1}{4}$ inch piece ginger, a few mint leaves, one small onion, salt, chilli powder and lime juice to taste. Grind all the ingredients with the exception of fish to paste. Apply on both the sides of fish. Put in a well-greased brown paper both the slices separately and tie up, steam the fish for ten minutes on each side.

Bed time

One cup skim milk.

On Gaining Weight

Strange as it may seem both the underweight and the overweight people are sufferers in their own way. Both suffer from an inferiority complex because the overweight people are too fat for comfort and the underweight people are too thin to look healthy. They look undernourished and starved and nothing seems to suit them.

The body can be compared to a furnace. Food in the form of fuel is fed into it and burned to produce heat and energy. In thin people the food is burnt uneconomically because either they are too active, hyper sensitive or over-anxious or nervous. Therefore, they have to take more food to compensate for this loss. But the weight-loser has to take in less food than her/his body needs to get along, thereby forcing the body to draw on stored up fat for the energy it requires. Now, you know why you have to eat more food because it is your job to take in more calories than are used up.

Small frequent meals rich in proteins, vitamins, carbohydrates and fats should be eaten by you. In addition to these you can also enjoy all the lovely foods that the fat people have to avoid such as ice creams, cakes and pudding and in between snacks. In the following pages is given a menu for seven days to be followed by all the weight-gainers. Besides, keep the few points mentioned below in mind if you are really interested in putting on weight.

1. Have three meals every day at regular hours. Start with a wholesome breakfast and have a healthy dinner and lunch. In between snacks are excellent for you but do not eat the sort of food that will kill your next regular meal, some of the preferable in-betweens are fruit juices, milk, fruits, cakes or ice creams.

2. If your appetite is weak, prepare foods tastefully and serve them attractively. But it is not easy to increase your appetite as it is not easy for the weight-losers to decrease their appetite but if you really want to fill your self up, you have got to eat. If necessary, 'use' some psychology on yourself. You can start by increasing the amount of food just slightly in the beginning. Then gradually you can increase the intake of your food and try to substitute high calorie foods for lower ones, all this will take time but you will surely come out a winner in the end.

3. Food should be easy on your teeth, chew properly and take your time to finish it, while having it relax yourself and enjoy it.

4. One of the most important factors in addition to diet is adequate rest and mental relaxation. A nap in the afternoon and a good sleep at night will not only help you to put on weight but will also make you look fresh and glowing. Also try to be relaxed at all times. If you are tense and worried most of the time, your digestive

system will not function properly. Exercise can help you to relax. Breathing is an easy and simple exercise. Lying on your back, breathe in slowly until your lungs can take in no more, pause for a second and expel the last vestige of breath through the open mouth. This will surely help you to relax—if nothing else will.

Seven-day Menu For Putting On Weight

FIRST DAY

Breakfast

Cashewnut omelette, toasts with generous amounts of butter, one banana, one cup milk.

Cashewnut omelette : Two eggs (beaten), handful of coriander leaves, few mint leaves, one green chilli (sliced), one medium tomato (sliced), eight fried cashewnuts (diced), four tablespoons grated cheese, salt to taste.

Place tomato, salt, mint, coriander leaves and chilli in a pan and cook till mixture turns soft. Remove from fire, cool and mix into eggs along with cashewnuts. Put two tablespoons butter on a girdle and pour the eggs into it. When both sides are done, sprinkle half cheese on the top, roll up and sprinkle with remainding cheese.

Mid-morning

One glass pineapple juice sweetened either with honey or glucose. (Pineapple juice contains an excellent digestive called bromelin.)

Lunch

Boiled rice, vegetable curry, sweet *raita*, *papad* and pickle (optional).

Vegetable curry : Take two tablespoons gram flour, $\frac{1}{4}$ teaspoon each of cumin, mustard and fenugreek seeds, $\frac{1}{4}$ teaspoon sliced ginger, pinch of asafoetida, a few curry leaves, $\frac{1}{2}$ teaspoon turmeric powder, two tablespoons tamarind water, 200 gram. mixed vegetables (tomatoes, potatoes, brinjals, lady fingers, cauliflower and french beans), one drumstick (scraped and diced), salt to taste, a few coriander leaves, two green chillis (minced). Heat two tablespoons ghee and toss in cumin seeds, mustard and fenugreek seeds, asafoetida, ginger and chillis. When the seeds stop crackling, put in the gram flour and fry to a golden colour. Put in two glasses of water, add all the vegetables with the exception of lady fingers. Put in the curry leaves and all the spices. When the vegetables are almost done, toss in the lady fingers and tamarind. Continue cooking till all the vegetables are done. Sprinkle corriander leaves on the top.

Sweet raita : one cup thick curd, one tablespoon each of finely sliced almonds and pistachios, a big pinch cardamom powder, a few drops essence of rose, sugar to taste.

Put the curd in a clean piece of cloth and tie loosely. Hang the bag for a couple of hours in order to enable all the liquid to drip through. Beat up with the help of a fork and mix in all the ingredints. Eat chilled.

Tea time

Hot chocolate.

Take $\frac{1}{4}$ cup water, two cups hot milk, two tablespoons chocolate or cocoa powder, two tablespoons whipped cream, a few drops essence of vanilla and sugar to taste. Heat water and melt the chocolate and sugar in it by stirring it nicely. Beat in the milk and essence. Serve topped with cream.

Dinner

Brain *korma*, poppy seed potatoes, buttered *roti*, carrot halva.

Brain *korma* : One brain (boiled), ½ teaspoon each of *garam masala* and powdered *shahjeera*, one medium tomato (sliced), ¼ teaspoon grated ginger, two flakes garlic, one small onion, a few coriander leaves, ¼ teaspoon turmeric powder, two green chillis (sliced), salt and chilli powder to taste. Grind ginger, garlic and onion to a paste. Heat two tablespoons *ghee* and add the paste and fry it to a pink colour. Add tomato, chillis and all the spices and cook till soft and dry. Add one cup hot water and put in the brain and corriander leaves. Cook for five minutes and remove from fire.

Poppy seed potatoes : One big potato (boiled and peeled), one tablespoon semolina or *sooji*, ½ tablespoon poppy seeds, salt, chilli and mango powder to taste. Cut the potato into thick slices about one-fourth inch thick. Dip in milk. Mix semolina with poppy seeds and spices, roll them in semolina mixture and shallow fry to a golden colour.

Carrot *halva* : Four tablespoons grated carrots, one cup milk, ¼ teaspoon cardamom powder, a few sliced nuts of your choice, sugar to taste. Put carrots in milk along with cardamom powder and cook till thick. Put in sugar and keep on stirring till it dissolves. Pour in two tablespoons *ghee* and fry till red. Sprinkle nuts on the top before eating.

Bed time

One cup hot milk with honey to induce sleep.

SECOND DAY

Breakfast

Meat omelette, one orange.

Meat omelette : Two eggs (beaten), three tablespoons boiled, minced mutton, a few sliced mint and coriander leaves, one small onion (minced), two green chillis (minced), ½ cup sliced spinach, two tablespoons cream, one tablespoon tomato ketchup, six fried bread squares. Heat one tablespoon oil and fry onion, chillis, coriander and mint leaves till soft. Add mutton and fry for five minutes, mix in the ketchcup and remove from fire. Steam the spinach and mix in the cream and one teaspoon of powdered cumin seeds. Add salt to beaten eggs. Fry the omelette in butter till set on both the sides, put mutton in the centre and fold over. Place the omelette in the centre of a plate, arrange spinach around it and eat with fried bread squares.

Mid-morning

One glass tomato juice.

Lunch

Dal delicious, buttered *roti*, mixed vegetable *raita*, brinjal *bharata*.

Dal delicious : Take ¼ cup *moong* dal, one medium tomato, ¼ teaspoon cumin seeds, ¼ teaspoon grated ginger, a few curry leaves, ¼ teaspoon turmeric powder, ½ teaspooon coarsely powdered coriander seeds, ¼ cup milk, one and a half tablespoons tomato ketchup, salt and chilli powder to taste. Boil *dal* in water till very soft, mash and pass through a fine sieve. Heat two tablespoons *ghee* and toss in cumin seeds, ginger and curry leaves. When the seeds stop popping, add tomato, all the spices and chilli and coriander leaves and cook till dry. Put in milk and ketchup and cook till smooth, add *dal* and the required amount of water and cook for five minutes more.

Mixed vegetable *raita* : 50 gram of mixed vegetables (carrot, cucumber, french beans, potato and peas), one cup curd, ¼ teaspoon grated ginger, one green chilli, (minced), ½ teaspoon roasted and ground cumin seeds, one tablespoon cream, salt, chilli powder and pepper to taste. Steam-cook all the vegetables with the exception of cucumber. Chop all the vegetables finely and mix with the rest of the above ingredients. Eat chilled.

Brinjal *bharata* : Take one deep purple brinjal, one medium onion, four flakes garlic, two green chillis (minced), ½ inch piece ginger, a handful of coriander leaves, one big tomato (sliced finely), ¼ teaspoon turmeric powder, ½ tablespoon coriander powder, ½ teaspoon ground cumin seeds, salt and chilli powder to taste, finely sliced onion, ginger and garlic. Roast brinjal on an open flame till the skin crinkles and turns completely black, toss in cold water and peel and dice into small pieces. Heat two tablespoons oil and fry onion, ginger and garlic till soft. Add tomato, chilli and all the spices and cook till the tomato turns soft, mix in the brinjals and cook for five minutes more. Sprinkle the corriander leaves on the top.

Tea time

Banana milk shake.

Banana milk shake : Take one ripe banana (mashed to a pulp), one cup chilled milk, ½ cup orange juice, sugar to taste, one stick vanilla ice cream. Put all the ingredients except ice cream in the blender and blend at high speed for one minute. Stir in ice cream and beat till smooth.

Dinner

Brown rice, *kheema* cutlets, spinach vegetable mix, finger chips, ice cream.

Brown rice : ½ cup rice, one medium onion, ½ inch piece ginger, one tablespoon coriander powder, ½ teaspoon *garam masala*, two cloves, one cardamon, one bay leaf, ¼ inch piece cinnamon stick, salt and chilli powder to taste. Wash rice and soak in water for one hour. Heat two tablespoons *ghee* and put in all the whole spices, add ginger and onion and fry till golden in colour. Add drained rice, salt, ground spices and enough water to stand one inch above the level of the rice. Cook till the rice is tender and dry.

Kheema cutlets : Take one cup minced mutton, 50 gram green peas, one small potato, a few mint leaves, a handful of coriander leaves, one green chilli, ½ inch piece ginger, one small onion, ½ teaspoon *garam masala*. salt and chilli powder to taste, one egg (beaten), one cup bread crumbs.

Boil meat in salted water along with peas and potato till tender and dry, then grind to a paste along with all the above ingredients with the exception of bread crumbs and eggs. Form into *patties*, roll in crumbs, dip in eggs, roll once again in crumbs and shallow fry to a golden colour.

Spinch vegetable mix : Take ½ cup spinach, one medium tomato, one green chilli, a handful of coriander leaves, ½ inch piece ginger, ½ teaspoon cumin seeds, ¼ teaspoon turmeric powder, 1 teaspoon coriander powder, ½ cup mixed sliced vegetables (pumpkin or marrow, potato, brinjal, french beans, carrots), salt and chilli powder to taste, one small onion. Heat two tablespoons *ghee* and toss in ginger and cumin seeds. When the seeds stop popping put in the onion and chilli and cook till soft. Put in the rest of the above ingredients with one cup water till the vegetables are cooked. Mash coarsely. Reheat before eating.

Bed time

One cup milk mixed with one tablespoon honey.

THIRD DAY

Breakfast

Western omelette, toast and butter.

Western omelette : Take two eggs, one tablespoon milk, ¼ cup grated cheese, a handful of coriander leaves, a few mint leaves, ¼ inch piece ginger, ½ tablespoon lime juice, two tablespoons grated coconut, a big pinch of sugar, one chilli, salt and chilli powder to taste. Grind together coconut, mint, coriander, ginger and sugar to a paste. Stir in lime juice and set aside. Beat the eggs with milk and salt. Melt two tablespoons butter in a pan and pour egg mixture into it. Cook until browned on both the sides. Cover half the omelette with half the cheese and with half the coconut mixture. Fold over and pour the rest of the coconut and cheese on top.

Mid-morning

Carrot cocktail.

Blend half cup carrot juice with half cup milk.

Lunch

Delightful *dal*, alu palak, mixed salad, buttered *roti*, one banana.

Delightful *dal*: Take ¼ cup black gram or urad *dal*, ¼ teaspoon cumin seeds, one small onion (sliced finely), one medium tomato (sliced finely), one green chilli (minced), ¼ teaspoon grated ginger, ¼ teaspoon turmeric powder, ½ teaspoon of *garam masala* and coriander powder, two tablespoons butter, a few mint leaves, salt and chilli powder to taste. Wash and soak *dal* in water for two hours and drain. Heat one tablespoon *ghee*, put in the *dal* and turmeric powder and enough water. When the *dal* turns tender and completely dry, remove from fire. Put in a serving dish and put powdered spices on the top. Heat one tablespoon *ghee* and toss in cumin seeds and ginger. When the seeds stop popping, put in the onion, chilli and tomato and cook for two minutes. Put over the *dal* along with butter and mint leaves.

Alu palak : Take ½ cup spinach, one medium potato (cubed), one medium white gourd or *tinda* (cubed), one big tomato (sliced), one small onion, ¼ teaspoon grated ginger, ¼ teaspoon turmeric powder, ½ teaspoon each of *garam masala* and coriander powder, salt and chilli powder to taste, one green chilli (minced). Heat two tablespoons *ghee* and fry onion and ginger till soft. Add potato and *tinda* and fry for a few minutes. Put in the spinach and tomato along with all the rest of the above ingredients. Mix well and then pour in ½ cup water. Remove when the vegetables are tender and a thick gravy is left.

Salad : Take raw vegetables of choice, mince them and season them with salt, pepper and lime juice.

Tea time

Curveous cocktail : ½ cup each of orange juice and milk, blend together and beat in one egg yolk and put honey to suit the taste. If you like you can also mix in one stick of vanilla ice cream.

Dinner

Boiled rice, tomato prawns, coriander potatoes, pudding.

Tomato prawns : 200 gram prawns (shelled and deviened), two medium tomatoes (sliced), one small onion, two flakes garlic, ¼ inch piece ginger, ½ cup coconut milk, ¼ teaspoon turmeric powder, one teaspoon each of coriander powder and ground cumin seeds, a handful of coriander leaves, salt and chilli powder to taste. Heat two tablespoons oil and fry onion, ginger and garlic till soft, put in the prawns and keep on frying till they stick to the bottom of the pan. Mix in the tomato along with the spices and salt. Put in the tomatoes and coconut milk and cook till the prawns are tender. Put coriander leaves on top.

Coriander potatoes : 100 gram baby potatoes, one medium tomato (sliced), ½ teaspoon *garam masala*, coriander powder and powdered cumin seeds, ¼ teaspoon pepper, 3 tablespoons finely chopped coriander leaves, salt and chilli powder to taste. Boil and peel the potatoes. Heat two tablespoons butter and fry the potatoes to a pale golden colour. Put in the tomato with spices and salt. Cook till the tomato turns soft and no gravy remains. Sprinkle coriander leaves on the top, mix well and remove from fire.

(Burnt sugar) pudding : Two tablespoons sugar, one well-beaten egg, one cup milk, a few drops essence of vanilla, a few sliced nuts of your choice. Put one tablespoon butter in a pan and put in the sugar. When the sugar dissolves and turns golden in colour, pour in the milk mixed with egg, vanilla and nuts. Cover the vessel with grease-proof paper and steam for half an hour or till the pudding is set.

Bed time

One cup milk mixed with one tablespoon honey.

FOURTH DAY

Breakfast

Fish omelette, toast, butter, one banana.

Fish omelette : Take four tablespoons boiled and flaked fish, two eggs, $\frac{1}{4}$ cup milk, one tablespoon flour, two tablespoons grated cheese, one tablespoon each of finely sliced onion and parsley, salt to taste, one chilli (minced). Beat the egg lightly. Stir in the rest of the ingredients. Melt two tablespoons butter in a hot frying pan and pour the mixture into it. Cook both the sides to a light golden colour. Eat with chilli sauce blended with tomato ketchup and, if you like, you can even have fingerchips with it.

Mid-morning

Spinach delight—½ cup carrot juice mixed with ½ cup spinach juice.

Lunch

Cauliflower queen, buttered *roti*, *rajmah.*

Cauliflower queen : Take 200 gram cauliflower (cut into flowerets), ½ teaspoon each of *garam masala* and powdered *shahjeera*, ¼ teaspoon each of powdered cardamoms and turmeric powder, ½ teaspoon grated ginger, one medium onion, six fried cashewnuts. one large tomato (sliced), a few coriander leaves, two tablespoons cream, salt and chilli powder to taste. Grind onion and ginger to a paste. Fry cauliflower flowerets to golden colour in *ghee* and drain. Heat two tablespoons *ghee* and fry onion paste to a golden colour. Add all the spices, salt and tomato and cook till soft and dry. Stir in the cream, cook till thick, put in the cauliflower and cashewnuts and half cup water and cook till no water is left. Put coriander leaves on the top before eating.

Rajmah : Take 50 gram *rajmah*, ¼ teaspoon grated ginger, 2 flakes garlic, one medium onion, one green chilli, a few each of mint and coriander leaves, one medium tomato, salt and chilli powder to taste, ½ teaspoon *garam masala*. Grind to a paste onion, ginger, garlic and chilli. Soak the beans in one cup boiling water for one hour, then boil in the water in which it was soaked. Heat two tablespoons *ghee* and fry the onion paste to a golden colour, add all the spices and tomato and cook till soft. Put in the *rajmah* along with the water in which it was boiled and cook till the gravy turns thick.

Tea time

Mango *phool.*

Take one medium raw mango, one glass milk, one cup water, sugar to taste, ¼ teaspoon powdered cardamoms, a pinch of saffron and crushed ice. Boil sugar and milk together, when the sugar dissolves, remove from fire and chill. Boil mango in water till soft and strain through a cloth. Chill mango pulp and mix with all the remaining ingredients.

Dinner

Chinese fried rice, chicken and sweet corn soup, fried cocktail prawns, Peking dush.

Chinese fried rice : Take one cup cooked rice, one egg (beaten), pinch of monsodium glutamate, one tablespoon shredded capsicum, a few cooked prawns, one green or spring onion (sliced) and salt to taste. Heat two teablespoons salad oil and fry the rice for five minutes. Mix in one teaspoon soya sauce, monsodium glutamate and salt. Remove from fire. Heat one tablespoon oil in a separate pan and fry onion and capsicum till soft. Add the prawns, mix well, then put in the egg and stir briskly till the egg breaks up in segments. Put in the rice`and mix thoroughly.

Chicken and sweet corn soup : Take 1½ cups chicken stock, ¼ cup canned and creamed corn, one egg (beaten), ½ teaspoon cornflour, two tablespoons boiled and shreded chicken, pinch of monsodium glutamate, salt to taste. Mix the cornflour with two tablespoons water to a paste. Heat chicken stock to boiling and mix in the corn and chicken, boil for a few minutes. Then add the rest of the ingredients with the exception of egg. Simmer over a gentle fire stirring all the time till the soup is slightly thickened. Remove from fire and add the beaten egg through a sieve to create thread-like shreds. Eat with soya and chilli sauce.

Fried cocktail prawns : Take 5 king-size prawns, two tablespoons cornstarch, one egg white, a pinch of monsodium glutamate, salt and pepper to taste. Beat egg white to a stiff froth and mix with one tablespoon cornstarch, salt and pepper and monsodium glutamate. Roll prawns in the remaining cornflour, dip in egg mixture and deep fry over a gentle fire to a golden brown colour.

Peking dush : Take four waterchestnuts or *shingara*, ½ cup cream, one orange (peeled and sliced), two tablespoons powdered sugar. Boil the chestnuts till soft. Peel and mash finely, mix in sugar and three-fourths of the cream. Chill nicely, pour remaining cream on the top and decorate with orange slices.

Bed time

One cup milk blended with one tablespoon honey.

FIPTH DAY

Breakfast

Missi roti, bowl of seasoned curd.

Missi roti : Take ¼ cup each of flour and gram flour, ¼ teaspoon grated ginger, one tiny onion (minced), a few sliced coriander leaves, one tiny tomato (sliced), one chilli (minced), salt and chilli powder to taste. Mix together all the above ingredients and add enough water to from a stiff dough. Roll into round *roti* or disc and shallow fry to a golden colour. Smear liberally with butter and eat with curd.

Mid-morning

Apple tonic consisting of one glass of apple juice.

Lunch

Boiled rice, pakoda curry, one banana, vegetable *tikki*.

Pakoda curry : Take one midium potato, one tiny onion (minced), one slice bread, pinch of soda bicarbonate, a few coriander leaves, ¼ teaspoon cumin seeds, ½ teaspoon crushed pomegranate seeds, one green chilli (minced), three tablespoons gram flour, one medium tomato (sliced), two tablespoons curd, ½ cup coconut milk, a few curry leaves, ¼ teaspoon turmeric powder, ¼ teaspoon *garam masala*, ½ teaspoon coriander powder, salt and chilli powder to taste. Mash the potato. Soak the slice of bread in water, squeeze dry and put into the potato along with chilli, coriander leaves, pomegranate seed and onion. Shape into small balls. Mix together gram flour, soda, salt and turmeric powder along with enough water to form a thick paste. Immerse the balls one by one into the *besan* paste and deep fry to a golden colour. To make the curry, melt one tablespoon butter and fry one medium onion and ½ teaspoon grated ginger to a golden colour. Add tomato along with all the spices, salt and curry leaves and curds and cook till dry. Add coconut milk along with ½ cup water. Bring to a boil, mix in the *pakodas* and boil for five minutes.

Vegetable *tikki :* Take 100 gram. mixed vegetables (french beans, peas, carrots, cabbage and potatoes); one tiny onion (minced), one green chilli (minced), two tablespoons gram flour, ½ teaspoon powdered cumin seeds, a handful of coriander leaves, a few mint leaves, salt and chilli powder to taste, ½ teaspoon grated ginger, ¼ teaspoon cumin seeds. Steam-cook all the vegetables and mash. Mix with the rest of the above ingredients and knead to a smooth mixture. Form into round *tikki* or cutlet and shallow fry to a golden colour.

Tea time

Orange soda.

Take one cup each of orange juice and milk, two cups soda, two sticks vanilla ice cream and sugar to taste. Mix together juices and sugar. Mix ice cream into soda and beat till it is partially dissolved. Mix in the milk mixture and take immediately.

Dinner

Stuffed fish in herbs, butter *roti*, Russian salad, fruit souffle.

Stuffed fish in herbs : Take one 250 gram. fish like pomfret, ½ cup each of coriander leaves and fenugreek leaves, one bunch green garlic, a few mint leaves, one tiny onion, one small tomato, ¼ teaspoon turmeric powder, ½ teaspoon each of coriander powder and powdered cumin seeds, salt and chilli powder to taste. Clean, scale and gut the fish. Make a slit in the centre of the fish and remove its centre bone carefully. Grind all the above ingredients to a coarse paste. Fill the fish with the stuffing and tie the fish up to keep the stuffing intact. Shallow fry to a golden brown colour.

Russian salad : Take one hard-boiled egg, 100 gram. mixed boiled vegetables (peas, carrots, potatoes, french beans and cucumber), one tinned pineapple slice (diced), ¼ cup mayonnaise sauce, two tablespoons cream. Mix all the above ingredients together and eat chilled. If you like, you can omit the egg.

Fruit souffle : Take 1½ slice of bread (trimmed and cut into pieces), one cup warm milk, one egg (beaten), two tablespoons butter, a few drops vanilla essence, ½ cup mixed diced fruits of your choice. Add sugar and butter to egg and whisk till frothy. Soak bread in milk and mix in the egg mixture and essence and fruit. Put in a greased souffie case and bake in preheated moderate oven. Serve topped with cream if you like.

Bed time

One cup milk mixed with one tablespoon honey.

SIXTH DAY

Breakfast

Vegetable *uppama*.

Vegetable *uppama :* 100 gram semolina or *suji*, ½ cup mixed, diced vegetables (carrots, peas, potatoes, beans and cabbage), one green chilli (minced); ½ teaspoon grated ginger, ¼ teaspoon mustard seeds, ¼ teaspoon each of *urad* and *chana dal*, a few curry leaves, a few fried cashewnuts, a handful of curry leaves. Salt to taste. Steam-cook all the vegatables. Heat one tablespoon *ghee* and fry the somolina to a light golden colour. Heat two tablespoons *ghee* and fry *dals* and mustard seeds to a red colour. Put in the ginger, chillies, curry leaves, salt and vegetables. Put in two cups water and bring to a boil. Add fried *rava*. Lower heat and keep on stirring till the mixture turns dry and thick. Mix in cashewnuts and coriander leaves. Serve with coconut chutney.

Coconut chutney : Take ¼ coconut, ½ inch ginger, ¼ cup coriander leaves, a few roasted grams, two green chillis, two tablespoons tamarind water, ¼ teaspoon each of mustard seeds and *urad dal*, a few curry leaves and salt to taste. Grind all the above ingredients to a paste with the exception of *dal*, mustard seeds and curry leaves. Fry in one teaspoon oil mustard seeds, *dal* and curry leaves till the *dal* turns red and put over the chutney.

Mid-morning

Cabbage cocktail: ½ cup of cabbage juice mixed with ¼ cup each of carrot and tomato juice.

Lunch

Boiled rice, potato *tikki*, fish curry, brinjal salad, one banana.

Potato *tikki* : Take 100 gram potatoes (boiled and peeled), a pinch of cumin seeds, one slice of bread.

Filling : One small onion (minced), a handful of coriander leaves, a few mint leaves, one green chilli (minced), salt and chilli powder to taste.

Soak bread in water and squeeze dry, mix into the potato along with salt and cumin seeds and knead to a smooth mixture. Mix all the filling ingredients together. Form the potatao mixture into rounds around a little of of the filling and shallow fry to a golden colour.

Fish curry : Take 250 gram fish (cut into slices), a medium onion, six flakes garlic, one big tomato (sliced), ¼ teaspoon turmeric powder, ½ teaspoon each of *gram masala* and coriander powder, two green chillis (minced), two tablespoons sour curd, a handful of coriander leaves, salt and chilli powder to taste. Clean and cut the fish into thin slices; apply salt and turmeric powder and set aside for half an hour. Fry fish lightly. Grind onion ginger and garlic to a paste. Heat two tablespoons oil and fry the paste to a golden colour. Add the spices, curd and tomato and cook till dry. Put in two cups water, bring to a boil, put in the slices of fish and cook till the fish is done. Sprinkle coriander leaves on top.

Brinjal salad : Take one medium brinjal, one tablespoon olive oil, one tablespoon lime juice, one small onion, one small tomato, one small capsicum and salt to taste. Cut onion, tomato and capscium into thin rings. Hold brinjal over an open flame till the skin turns completely black. Skin brinjal while still hot and put in bowl with olive oil, lime juice and salt. Beat to a smooth mixture, would into a form of brinjal and decorate with the remaining raw vegetables.

Tea time

Hot chocolate.

Dinner

Egg *bhurji*, Punjabi alu, mixed vegetable *raita*, buttered *roti*, burnt sugar pudding.

Egg *bhurji* : Take two well-beaten eggs, four tablespoons shelled peas, and medium tomato (diced), one small onion (minced), two green chillis (minced), a few coriander leaves, salt and pepper to taste. Boil the peas. Heat one tablespoon *ghee* and fry onion till red, put in the chillis, coriander leaves, tomato and salt cook till soft. Put in the peas and cook till dry, then add the eggs and keep on stirring till firm.

Punjabi *alu* : Take two medium potatoes (boiled, peeled and diced), ½ cup curd, one green chilli (minced), ¼ teaspoon grated ginger, a few coriander leaves, ½ teaspoon each of *garam masala* and coriander powder and salt and chilli powder to taste. Fry the potatoes to golden brown colour. Put the fried potatoes in a pan along with the rest of the above ingredients and keep on stirring till the curd turns brown.

Bed time

One cup milk mixed with one tablespoon honey.

SEVENTH DAY

Breakfast

Meat omelette, toast and butter.

Mid-morning

One glass grape juice.

Lunch

Boiled rice, palak alu, one cup curd, one apple, meat *kofta* curry,

Meat *kofta* curry : For *kofta*—150 gram ground mutton, boiled in salted water, one tiny onion, one green chilli, ¼ teaspoon *garam masala*, ½ slice bread, ¼ teaspoon grated ginger, a few each of coriander and mint leaves and salt to taste. For curry—one medium onion, two flakes garlic, ¼ teaspoon grated ginger, teaspoon coriander seeds, one clove, one small piece cinnamon stick, one cardamon, ¼ teaspoon *shahjeera* one teaspoon poppy seeds, two green chillis, a handful of corriander leaves, $\frac{1}{2}$ teaspoon turmeric powder, one medium tomato, two tablespoons grated coconut, one cup thin and $\frac{1}{2}$ cup thick coconut milk and salt and chilli powder to taste.

Grind onion, ginger, garlic, poppy seeds, chillis and all the spices to a paste. On the stone, grind all the *kofta* ingredients to a paste with the exception of bread. Soak the bread in water, squeeze dry and add to the ground meat mixture. Form into small balls and deep fry to a golden brown colour. Heat two tablespoons *ghee* and fry the remaining ground *masala* nicely. Add tomatoes and cook till they turn soft. Add thin milk and turmeric powder. Bring to a boil, reduce heat and toss in the *koftas*. Cook for five minutes, put in the thick milk bring to simmering point and remove from fire.

Tea time

Banana cream shake.

Dinner

Buttered *roti*, prawn *masala* fry, butter *dal*, flaming banana dessert, mixed vegetable salad.

Prawn *masala* fry : Take 15 prawns (cleaned, shelled and deviened), one big onion, a small piece of coconut, two flakes garlic, $\frac{1}{8}$ teaspoon turmeric powder, a few coriander leaves, one teaspoon cumin seeds, $\frac{1}{2}$ inch piece cinnamon stick, two cloves and salt and chilli powder to taste.

Powder together all the spices. Apply turmeric and salt to prawns and set aside for one hour. Heat three tablespoons oil and put in all the above ing edients with the exception of coconut. Cover tightly and cook over a slow fire till the mixture turns dry. Add coconut and keep on stirring till the mixture turns golden. Sprinkle coriander leaves on top.

Butter *dal* : Take 50 gram. *urad dal,* ⅓ cup milk, two tablespoons cream, one tablespoon white unsalted butter, ½ teaspoon turmeric powder, one teaspoon raisins, ½ teaspoon cumin seeds, and salt and chilli powder to taste, a few sliced nuts. Fry the nuts and raisins. Soak the *dal* in water for one hour. Put along with water in which it was soaked in a pan. Add milk and turmeric powder. Cover and cook over a medium fire till the *dal* is done and practically no water is left, put in cream and if you like one tablespoon tomato ketchup. Mix well and remove from fire. Put on the top nuts, butter and raisins.

Flaming banana dessert : Take two peeled bananas (halved), two tablespoons butter, two tablespoons dry coconut. Sugar to taste. A big pinch nutneg, ½ teaspoon ground cardamoms and three tablespoons rum. Melt butter, add bananas and sprinkle half of the sugar and spices on the top. Cook over a slow fire till the bananas are lightly brown on the underside. Turn over remaining sugar and spices and cook till all the sides are light brown. Put in a heat-proof glass dish, pour three tablespoons whipped cream on the top. Sprinkle coconut on the whole. Heat rum and pour over the bananas. Touch lighted match to the rum and carry ablaze to the table.

Bed time

On cup milk mixed with one tablespoon honey.

□ □ □

Also in Orient Paperbacks

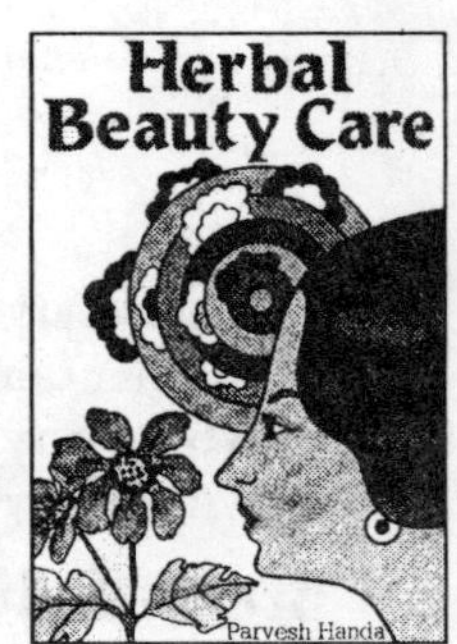

Herbal Beauty Care

Parvesh Handa

Parvesh Handa, the well known beautician and columnist, gives hundreds of recipes for every kind of beauty preparation — cleansing creams and face masks. Conditioners for your hands, neck, feet and knees, washing scrubs, lotions and oils for bath and for massage, skin tonics, antiwrinkle creams, astringents, moisturisers and toners, shampoos, hair conditioners and colourants, deodarants and powders — all based on fruits, vegetables, herbs and spices. There are honey, curd, milk, lemon, vinegar and such other things to help you be a beautiful woman. And a chapter on simple exercises and diets based on nature foods to keep you fresh and trim.

"The book meets the burgeoning demand for cosmetics made of herbs and such things."

Amrita Bazar Patrika

"Provides recipes for skin care, for the core of the body, eyes, teeth, hair, face, etc... contains useful information on the properties of some common herbs and ingredients."

Pioneer

Illustrated | pp 160 | Rs. 70.00

Also in Orient Paperbacks

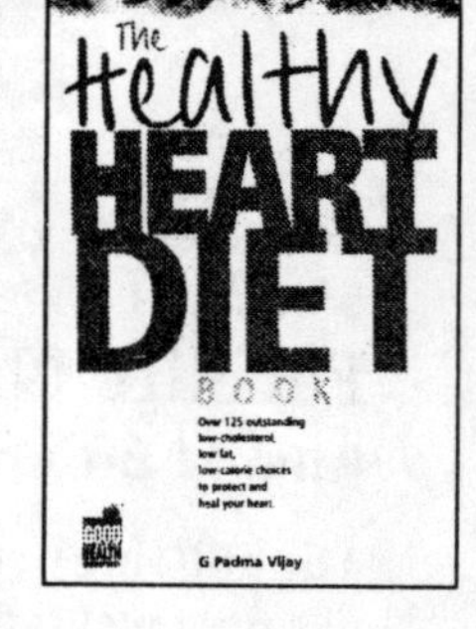

The Healthy Heart Diet Book

G Padma Vijay

Over 125 outstanding low-cholesterol, low fat, low-calorie choices to protect and heal your heart.

Foods are the first line of defence against heart disease. You can greatly reduce your risk of developing heart disease or having a heart attack by keeping track of how much you eat. And what you eat. It is a matter of choice. Your choice.

A healthy selection of foods is not limited to persons challenged with heart problems. It is for everyone. Only that for people with heart disease the choice of food is more critical. It is their lifeline.

Easy-to-read. Easy-to-follow. The book clearly explains the things you need to do to have a healthy heart.

pp 192 | Rs. 150.00

Also in Orient Paperbacks

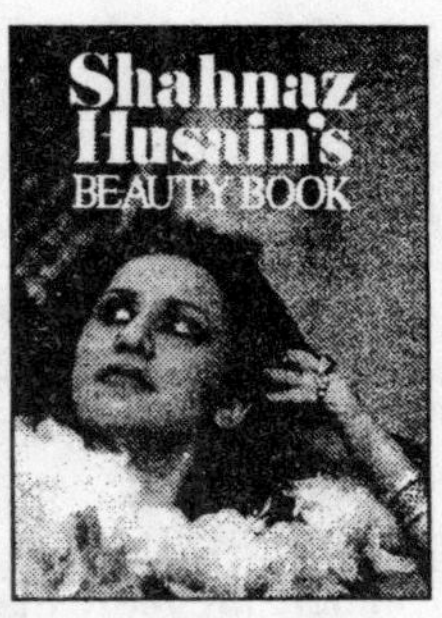

Shahnaz Husain's Beauty Book

"Internationally famous — she is an established name in Skin and Hair care."

The New York Times

"She is spreading the rich herbal heritage of India around the world."

Guardian

"Fabulous and fascinating."

Barbara Cartland, London

"Shahnaz Husain combines ancient herbal remedies with scientific techniques very effectively."

Washington Post, USA

"Shahnaz Husain is India's sacred goddess of beauty."

Jardin Desmodes, Paris

"Internationally recognized authority on herbs... a Phenomenal success."

B.B.C.

26 Colour Pic. | Illustrated | pp 184 | Rs. 195.00

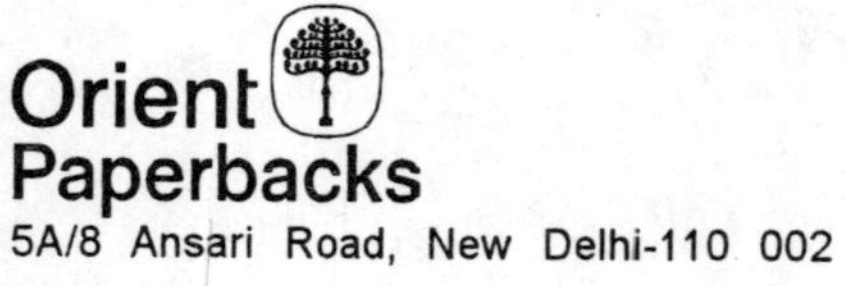
Orient
Paperbacks
5A/8 Ansari Road, New Delhi-110 002